Natural
Remedies
for Inflammation

Natural Remedies
for Inflammation

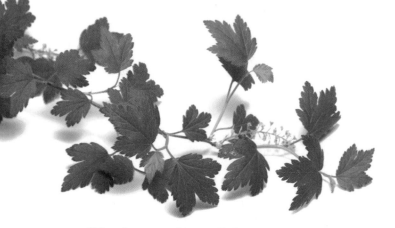

Christopher Vasey, N.D.

Translated by Jon E. Graham

Healing Arts Press
Rochester, Vermont • Toronto, Canada

Healing Arts Press
One Park Street
Rochester, Vermont 05767
www.HealingArtsPress.com

Healing Arts Press is a division of Inner Traditions International

Originally published in French under the title *Les anti-inflammatoires naturels: Prévenir et guérir de façon naturelle* by Éditions Jouvence, www.editions-jouvence.com, info@editions-jouvence.com
First U.S. edition published in 2014 by Healing Arts Press

Note to the reader: This book is intended as an informational guide. The remedies, approaches, and techniques described herein are meant to supplement, and not to be a substitute for, professional medical care or treatment. They should not be used to treat a serious ailment without prior consultation with a qualified health care professional.

Library of Congress Cataloging-in-Publication Data
Vasey, Christopher.
  [Anti-inflammatoires naturels. English]
  Natural remedies for inflammation / Christopher Vasey, N.D.; translated by Jon E. Graham. — First U.S. edition.
       pages cm
  Includes index.
    ISBN 978-1-62055-323-7 (paperback) — ISBN 978-1-62055-324-4 (e-book)
  1. Inflammation—Alternative treatment. 2. Inflammation—Diet therapy. 3. Alternative medicine. I. Title.
  RB131.V3713 2014
  616′.0473—dc23
                                                                      2014015422

Printed and bound in Canada by Friesens

10 9 8 7 6 5 4 3 2

Text design and layout by Virginia Scott Bowman
This book was typeset in Garamond Premier Pro and Gill Sans with Rotis Sans and Suomi Sans used as display typefaces
Anatomical drawings by Rosalie Vasey

To send correspondence to the author of this book, mail a first-class letter to the author c/o Inner Traditions • Bear & Company, One Park Street, Rochester, VT 05767, and we will forward the communication, or contact the author directly at **www.christophervasey.ch/anglais/home.html**.

Contents

✍

PART ONE

The Inflammation Syndrome

Anti-inflammatory drugs are the bestselling pharmaceutical products on the market. Not only are the number of inflammatory diseases increasing, but they afflict more and more people with ever increasing severity. Anti-inflammatory drugs such as aspirin and cortisone are powerful and effective. They are accompanied by many contraindications, though, which makes their use potentially hazardous.

It is therefore worth knowing that nature offers us a host of medicinal plants, as well as other remedies, with anti-inflammatory effects. Their greatest benefit is that they can be used with no harmful side effects. However, natural medicine does not limit itself to fighting the symptoms but addresses the cellular terrain that permitted those symptoms to appear in the first place. In fact, its primary focus is to remove the cause of the illness, and its treatment of the symptoms is only a secondary concern. The activities of the anti-inflammatory agents it uses are consequently supported by a profound correction of the terrain as the basis of the treatment.

The issues of cellular terrain restoration and the destruction of the germs responsible for the bulk of inflammations will not be dealt with here, as I have already covered this subject in some depth in my previous books, especially those pertaining to detoxification.

The purpose of this book is to present inflammation from the point of view of natural medicine, to restore it to its proper place in the general context of the body's defense mechanisms, and to offer a selection of safe and natural anti-inflammatory substances. They can be used, for simple ailments, by individuals treating their problems personally, but in serious disorders, and if individuals have any cause for concern, it is imperative that they seek the advice of a trained professional.

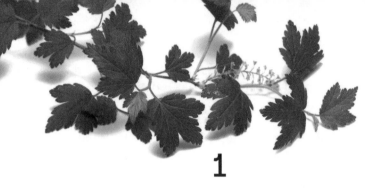

1

The Body's Defenses

Inflammation Reactions

The efforts undertaken by the body to protect itself against an irritating or aggressive agent (such as a germ or poison) are often accompanied by painful and annoying inflammation. The vast majority of patients would gladly do without this problem. However, inflammation does not merely accompany the body's defensive reactions; it is itself part of the body's defense system. This is why we can talk of an "inflammatory reaction" when describing it—to show the useful, active nature of the role inflammation plays in protecting the body. We cannot do without it.

To truly grasp what inflammation is, we need to deal with three major questions:

1. Why does the body need to defend itself?
2. What is attacking the body?
3. How does the body defend itself?

WHY DOES THE BODY
NEED TO DEFEND ITSELF?

The body employs different procedures to defend itself; their main purpose is to protect the cells of the body, but the body also looks to protect those cells' environment: the terrain.

The Cells of the Human Body

The human body is an extremely complex object made up of some fifty billion cells. These come in different varieties depending on the organ or part of the body to which they belong. Each one has its specific task to perform, but it does this in accord with the logic that oversees the entire body. It conforms, or, more exactly, submits, to the will of the whole. This is essential, as the proper functioning of the entire body and its survival depends on this compliance.

This collection of cells that forms our body is incapable of tolerating in its midst the presence of foreign cells, whose behavior conflicts with the body's overall harmony.

Out of all the foreign cells that enter the body, the majority are "killed." This is the case with the cells belonging to the foods we eat. They are broken down into smaller particles that are integrated into our tissues. For example, the cells of a vege-

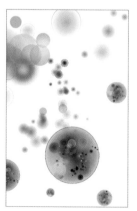

The human body consists of some fifty billion cells.

table or a piece of meat do not survive in their original composition. Cooking and the digestive process divide them into simple elements (amino acids, vitamins, and so on), which will then be integrated into the physical structure of the body or used as fuel.

A portion of the cells that enter our bodies are not killed (or not all at once). These are germs—that is, bacteria, fungi, molds, and parasites. Some of these integrate perfectly into the overall functioning of the body, such as those that restore the intestinal flora. The characteristics of others do not permit their harmonious integration into the body. They play no role in maintaining the general well-being of the body but live, in accordance with their own needs, at the expense and to the detriment of the whole. They are a threat to the body's proper functioning and sometimes even its very survival. The body therefore has to react against these invaders in order to protect itself.

The Terrain

Discussion of the cells alone could give a false or overly fragmentary vision of the body. We must also speak of the environment in which the cells live, in other words the terrain. This environment is liquid and consists of four different kinds of fluids:

1. **Blood** is familiar to everyone. It circulates through the vascular network, in other words the arteries, veins, and blood capillaries. This liquid represents 5 percent of total body weight.

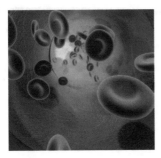

The blood represents 5 percent of the body's weight.

2. **Extracellular fluid** surrounds and bathes the exterior of the cells. It fills the tiny spaces that separate one cell from the next. It forms the external environment of the cells, the vast ocean in which they are immersed. This extracellular fluid is whitish in color. It is derived from blood plasma, which is the fluid part of blood, minus the red blood cells.

3. **Lymph** circulates in the lymph vessels. It is basically the same as extracellular fluid and its color is also whitish. Lymph removes some of the toxins produced by the cells and transports them into the bloodstream. In fact, the lymph vessels discharge their cargo into the blood network at the level of the subclavian veins. Lymph and extracellular fluid together account for 15 percent of total body weight.

4. **Intracellular fluid** is the liquid located inside the cells. Given the fact that cells are so small that they cannot be seen by the naked eye, their individual volume is extremely tiny. However, when added all together, these spaces form a fairly large volume. In fact, it is so large that intracellular fluid accounts for 50 percent of total body weight. This fluid is whitish in color and its composition is quite similar to that of extracellular fluid.

All of these fluids together make up the body's terrain and account for 70 percent of the body's total weight. The cells are entirely dependent on these fluids. They carry the nutrients (such as oxygen, minerals, and amino acids) the cells need to function. These same fluids transport the wastes or toxins expelled by the cells to the eliminatory organs—the liver, intestines, kidneys, skin, and lungs—to be eliminated from the body.* The cells' very survival is thus dependent on these fluids. If they do not supply the cells with all the nutrients they require, the

---

*See my earlier books on detoxification such as *Optimal Detox: How to Cleanse Your Body of Colloidal and Crystalline Toxins* (Rochester, Vt.: Healing Arts Press, 2013).

cells will weaken to the point that they can no longer perform their work properly. If they are saturated with wastes, they will be suffocated and attacked by the poison these wastes contain.

There is, therefore, an ideal composition for the body's cellular terrain that guarantees its cells an optimal environment for functioning. It so happens that every substance that enters the terrain alters its composition and thereby influences the cells' state of health positively or adversely. This influence will be beneficial if the substance can be integrated into the body—in other words, if it can find its proper place in the body's organization and structure. In the opposite case, the substance's influence will be negative and the cells will be endangered. This will then force the body to react more or less forcefully according to the danger posed by the invader, in order to neutralize or eliminate it.

WHAT IS ATTACKING THE BODY?

Countless invaders capable of provoking a defensive reaction from the body exist. They can be divided into four groups, based on their origin.

Microbial Invaders

Germs (in other words, bacteria, viruses, and yeasts) are living entities with their own functional logic. They therefore have no place in the human body, as they will be foreign guests who disturb its functioning (with the exception of the bacteria making up the intestinal flora). By setting up shop and multiplying in the body, they attack it in a variety of ways.

While some germs can live in the hollow organs like the intestines or bladder, others find favorable living conditions only inside the cells. In order to enter them, they release enzymes that attack the cellular membrane. The destruction of even a tiny bit of this surface will allow them to penetrate it. Once inside, they release other enzymes that carve up the large molecules

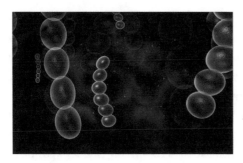

Streptococcus bacteria are one of the causes of pneumonia.

surrounding them into pieces small enough for them to assimilate. In this way they destroy the nucleus, the organelles, and the cytoplasm of the cell.

When an infection occurs, though, it is not simply one germ at work but thousands of similar germs attacking entire tissues. This can result in lesions of varying size, which will disrupt the functioning of the organ to which the cells belong, which will in turn cause dysfunction in the entire body.

Germs also attack the body through the toxins they produce. As living entities germs (with the exception of viruses) produce wastes and metabolic residues as a normal consequence of their functioning. They expel these wastes into their immediate environment, in other words the tissues.

It so happens that some of these substances are toxic to human beings, even in the minimal quantities in which they are produced in these circumstances. Because they are carried by the bloodstream to other regions of the body, they cause damage not only to their immediate surroundings but to fairly distant regions as well. The degree of their toxicity is not uniform; some have mild effects, while others can be quite devastating.

Chemical Invaders

There are two kinds of chemical substances that enter our bodies. Some are physiologically necessary, and the body integrates them. Others do not fulfill any physiological requirements, and the body has no way of integrating them into its normal biological cycles. When these chemicals get in, they disrupt and endanger the body's proper functioning. In this case we are dealing not with germs, which are living entities, but with various molecular substances that, through their natural properties, attack the body.

Among these chemical invaders, we can include the substances from the plant and animal kingdoms that are called "poisonous" or "toxic" because of the ill effects they produce in the body. These can be snake venom, the venom of bees, wasps, and other insects, poisonous mushrooms, and toxic plants. Other groups of chemical invaders have diverse origins. They include, among others, the heavy metals found in polluted air, ground, and water; drugs and vaccines; and agricultural products like insecticides and herbicides.

Individuals with allergies also have to contend with allergens (pollen, dust, certain foods, and so on), which are also potential invaders capable of triggering a defensive inflammatory reaction.

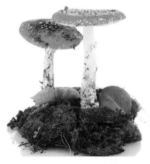

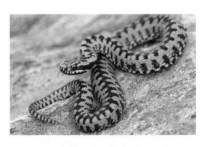

*Viper venom
is another chemical invader.*

*Red amanita is included
among the list of toxic
chemical invaders.*

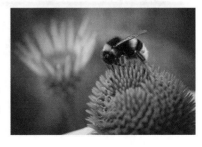

*Allergens like pollen can trigger
the body's use of inflammation
as a defense mechanism.*

THE INVADERS OF THE BODY

- Germs
- Poisons
- Foreign bodies
- Toxins

Physical Invaders

Various foreign bodies can find their way into the body. Because they are foreign, the body has to adopt a defensive stance toward them. Some of them find entry from the outside. These would be the splinters that are pushed into our skin—small pieces of wood, rose thorns, sea urchin spines, or metal particles (bomb shrapnel during armed conflict, for example). Another group comes from inside the body. This is the case, for example, with serious joint afflictions. As the tissues deteriorate, pieces of cartilage or bone become detached. Their presence between the contact surfaces of the two bones in the joint will create lesions and an inflammatory reaction.

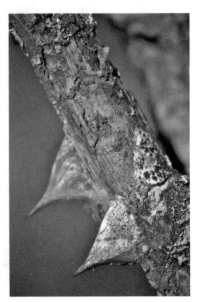

The body must defend itself when pricked by a rose thorn.

The body's own dead cells can also represent a threat when they suddenly collect in too large a number in the tissues. Cells are constantly dying and the body is always ridding itself of them. Sometimes an excessive number of cells are killed or destroyed. The resulting mass of dead cells exceeds the body's elimination capacity, and they become a threat.

Trauma is the usual cause of this kind of buildup of an excessive number of dead cells. A violent blow on any part of the body will crush and destroy the cells there. A similar situation occurs when tissues are destroyed by a major burn, whether it is due to heat, ionizing radiation (radiation therapy or atomic blast), or, quite simply, overexposure to the sun.

Toxins

Toxins are the waste products that result from the body's normal functioning. In small quantities they are quite tolerable. In the opposite case, however, they are an assault on the body. These toxins come primarily from the foods we eat. Proteins, for example, produce uric acid, urea, and creatinine, while fats produce saturated fatty acids and cholesterol. And many foods produce acidic toxins: white sugar creates pyruvic acid, bread produces phytic acid, fats produce acetoacetic acid, and so forth. Stimulants like coffee, tea, cocoa, alcohol, and tobacco also contribute to the supply of toxins.

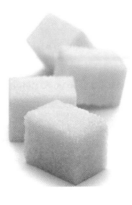

The pyruvic acid of sugar produces numerous toxins.

When people overeat their bodies receive more nutritive substances than they require, and hence a portion of them are not used. Although they are nutrients, they pose a burden to the terrain, and therefore they can be regarded as toxins. Furthermore, by fermenting or putrefying in the intestines, foods produce numerous poisons (skatoles, indoles, phenols, ptomaine, et cetera) that are all toxins poisoning the body.

The presence of a certain amount of toxins in the body is perfectly normal. The body is equipped to get rid of them. They do not pose any threat to it as long as they are present only in small quantities. Unfortunately, in our current era of overeating, the production of toxins exceeds the capacities of the eliminatory organs (the liver, intestines, kidneys, skin, and lungs).

Some toxins are not aggressive or irritating in nature. When they are present in large number, they are merely an annoying burden that causes congestion in the organs. Others are aggressive and irritating. In normal concentration levels in the terrain, they will not injure the cells. But when their number increases, their corrosive, irritating nature will make itself fully felt. This is when they will attack and inflame the tissues.

Gout, for example, is an inflammation of the big toe caused by an excess of uric acid, a toxin produced during the digestion of certain foods. Many eczema outbreaks are caused by an excess of acids supplied by the foods ingested by the individual, whose body seeks to eliminate them through perspiration. An overload of starch residues on the bronchial tubes can cause them to become inflamed even when not a single germ is present.

All terrain with a severe overload of toxins will be subject to a range of irritation that is capable of manifesting in inflammation of those organs that are having an increasingly difficult time coping with the toxic burden.

HOW DOES THE BODY DEFEND ITSELF?

The fundamental problem faced by a body whose defense system has been triggered is the presence of harmful elements (toxins, poisons, germs, allergens). Its major objective will therefore be to eliminate them in order to save itself.

It is common knowledge that the body is constantly striving to rid itself of anything that poses a threat to its functioning and survival. The body's five eliminatory organs—the liver, intestines, kidneys, skin, and lungs—continuously filter wastes and poisons out of the bloodstream. These noxious substances are subsequently expelled in the form of bile, stools, urine, sweat, and exhaled air.

This elimination labor—which is a defense mechanism—manifests much more intensely when the level of harmful elements is raised to excessive proportions. It can take very visible, even spectacular forms whose eliminatory purpose often goes unrecognized.

This involves all classes of illness: pimples, bronchitis, hives, coughs, and so on. In allopathic medicine they are each considered separate pathological states with different causes and characteristics. In natural medicine they are all believed to have one

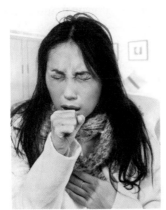

Coughing allows the body to get rid of excess wastes that are harmful to the body.

cause as their common source—the accumulation of toxins—and to exhibit the same effort—that undertaken by the body to eliminate the wastes and toxins that threaten its health. Their different characteristics are simply a result of the different areas in which the reaction takes place.

Because of their preeminently eliminatory nature, natural medicine regards diseases as first and foremost cleansing and detoxification crises.

The fundamentally eliminatory nature of diseases is easy to observe. With illnesses affecting the respiratory tract, for example, the elimination of toxins (accompanied sometimes by an infection) is diagnosed as sinusitis when they occur in the sinuses, as a cold when in the nose, as a sore throat when in the pharynx, as bronchitis when in the bronchial tubes, and so on. The general impression is that these are diseases with no common factors, insofar as each has its own name. However, they are all manifestations of the efforts undertaken by the body to get rid of an accumulation of wastes and poisons, whose presence is a threat to its continued good health.

If the body is constantly defending itself by trying to rid itself of the harmful elements threatening it, the visible manifestations of its activity will differ over the course of time. They will vary in accordance with the shifting balance of power between the invaders (toxins, germs, poisons) and what is being invaded (the body).

The process of the body's defenses can be broken down into four major stages.

THE FOUR STAGES
OF THE BODY'S DEFENSES

Over the course of the first two steps, the intensity of the body's defensive reaction increases, while the final two stages are characterized by a reduction of intensity.

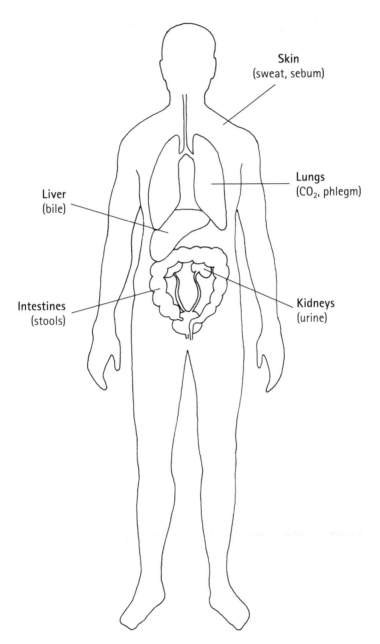

Skin
(sweat, sebum)

Lungs
(CO_2, phlegm)

Liver
(bile)

Intestines
(stools)

Kidneys
(urine)

The five eliminatory organs for ridding the body of toxins

THE FOUR STAGES OF THE BODY'S DEFENSE SYSTEM	
Nature of the Reaction	**Type of Illness**
Weak	Feeling poorly
Acute	Acute illness
Chronic	Chronic disease
Absence of any reaction	Degenerative disease

1. Weak Reaction (Feeling Poorly)

The body is troubled by elements of one kind or another. Their concentration and harmful nature are minimal. The drawbacks caused by their presence are not important enough to trigger a sharp reaction. The body does react, but weakly. This is when temporary states of indisposition appear, such as uncustomary nervous tension, insomnia, headaches, and so forth. These are all alarm signals indicating that disruptive influences have appeared and the body is beginning to fight them. We are not yet at the stage of illnesses, strictly speaking; we are simply at a stage where we are ailing or feeling poorly.

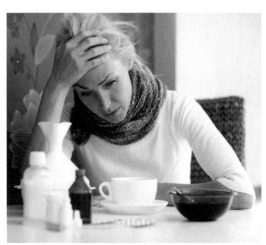

A headache is an alarm bell warning of a disruption in the body.

If nothing is done to remove the causes of disorder, they will increase. The body will then be forced to react more vigorously, as can be seen in the next stage.

2. Acute Reaction (Acute Illness)

At this stage the level of disruptive foreign substances has increased to such an extent that the body's tolerance level has been exceeded. It is no longer able to tolerate this presence and reacts vigorously against it. The body takes energetic steps to neutralize, destroy, and eliminate the elements endangering it. All the body's vital forces are mobilized to expel the intruders. This results in an overall acceleration of metabolism and defense mechanisms. These efforts manifest in visible ways: skin eruptions, the formation of abscesses, runny nose, diarrhea, urine charged with toxins, profuse sweating, and so on.

Allopathic medicine regards these defensive reactions as distinct diseases. Natural medicine, however, looks at them as cleansing crises caused by the body itself in reaction against a disruptive element.

Acute cleansing crises—or acute illnesses—are characteristically violent. The fever that accompanies them is evidence of the intense energy deployed by the body to protect itself. They are also of short duration. This intense effort allows a rapid return to normalcy.

3. Chronic Reaction (Chronic Disease)

When acute reactions have not achieved their goal, the body must continue its efforts in the chronic mode. As the harmful elements have not been neutralized and eliminated, they remain stagnant in the terrain, forcing the body to repeat its efforts over time. The level of reactive incidences will increase in proportion to the arrival of new toxins.

The body's defense system is now being called upon repeatedly, as it is never able to achieve its goal. While it does manage

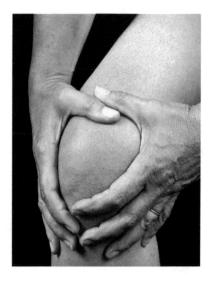

Chronic joint pain can result from chronic activation of the body's defense system.

to eliminate some of the toxins, it can never get rid of them all. Those toxins that remain are continually being bolstered by the new ones that continue to arrive. When they combine they again exceed the body's tolerance threshold and trigger a new reaction by its defenses. This is why we often see repeated outbreaks of eczema, asthma attacks, or joint pain every few months.

Another cause of chronic ailments is the continuous arrival of disruptive agents (such as toxins or germs) in the body. Their recurring contribution compels the body to react regularly, hence chronically. For example, excessive consumption of foods that produce uric acid causes joint inflammations like gout, that of acidifying foods causes sciatica and neuritis, that of foods rich in starch and sugar causes discharges by the respiratory tract.

Whereas in the previous stage the body's defensive reactions were violent and short, the chronic reactions here are generally less intense and persist over longer periods of time.

4. Absence of Reaction (Degenerative Disease)
The body's defensive reactions require an expenditure of energy. When the body's energy reserves are constantly being

drawn on, as is the case with chronic diseases, they will eventually shrink and vanish. The body can therefore reach a point where it no longer has enough strength to react. It is no longer capable of destroying and eliminating the noxious elements attacking it.

Every kind of disorder becomes possible when this stage is reached. Cellular life progressively deviates from its norm, and the organic life becomes increasingly disorganized. This is exhibited by the destruction of certain tissues or organs (sclerosis, irreversible lesions, deformations), by aberrant cell behaviors (cancer), or by the body's inability to defend itself as an organized whole against invasions by germs or viruses (AIDS, various immune system deficiencies). The stage of degenerative diseases has now been reached. The invader has not been destroyed but is now in a good position to destroy and disrupt the body.

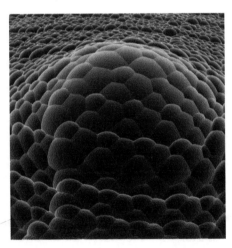

Degenerated cell: the organic life is disorganized.

These diseases are characterized by their lack of intensity (heat and strength) and by their duration. While in the preceding three stages the body could still defend itself, in this final phase it can no longer do so, or at best it can do so only weakly, which can lead to all manner of excesses and degeneration.

THE INFLAMMATORY REACTION

The inflammatory reaction belongs to the second stage, that of acute reactions by the body's defenses. In fact, this defense mechanism is intensely powerful; it could even be described as violent. Normally it is of short duration, though under certain circumstances it can become chronic. When this happens it enters the third stage. But let's look at the details.

At the level of the defense system's acute reactions of the second stage, the body can respond in one of two ways. One is global, because it involves the entire body. The other is local, as it is limited to a well-defined part of the body; this is the inflammatory reaction.

The Global Reaction

This reaction consists of an overall acceleration of physiological functions for the purpose of neutralizing and eliminating harmful elements. The eliminatory organs intensify their labor of filtering the bloodstream and expelling toxins. This results in an acceleration of intestinal transit, sometimes to the point of diarrhea; the urine is more heavily charged with wastes, the lungs expel greater quantities of phlegm, skin eruptions occur, and night sweats appear, as does increased perspiration during the day.

The destruction of toxins by oxidation and the good functioning of the eliminatory organs requires an increased intake of oxygen, which leads to an increase in the rhythm of breathing. This acceleration automatically causes an acceleration of the cardiac rhythm and the circulation of the bloodstream. Cellular exchanges and combustions also intensify. All these reactions produce heat, which leads to a heightened body temperature, better known as fever.

The Local Reaction

Instead of taking place in the whole body, the defensive reaction can involve only a limited, well-defined area of the body. The defensive reactions concentrate on this region to prevent a localized invader from affecting the rest of the body. Toxins are not usually targeted by a localized response; because they are more or less evenly distributed in the tissues, they require a global response. The targeted response is aimed at invaders that are few in number, powerful, and confined to a single area, such as germs or poisonous substances that enter the body.

THE INFLAMMATORY REACTION		
	Global Reaction	**Local Reaction**
Field of Action	Whole body	Limited region of the body
Invaders	Toxins and germs	Germs, chemical and physical invaders
Metabolisms	Overall acceleration	Local acceleration

In the case of local reactions, there can be an immune or inflammatory response.

The immune reaction is very precise and efficient. The immune system carefully analyzes the nature of the invader in order to implement the best adapted defense possible. It begins by detecting the precise location of the invader and then works to determine its different characteristics in order to identify its weaknesses. Then, based on the data it has received, the immune system will activate the production of white blood cells specially equipped to destroy the invader.

While the immune system of defense is quite effective, its main drawback is that it requires time to be properly implemented. The detection and analysis of the invader, and then the production of targeted white blood cells, are processes that take

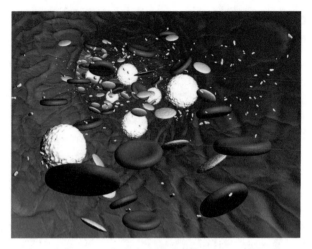

The production of white blood cells requires a certain amount of time before they can form an operational defense system.

time. A full preparation must be performed before the immune defense system can go into operation. During this time the invader—a poison or a germ, for example—can cause serious damage. When germs are involved, they can get established and multiply extensively before the defense system is able to interrupt their activity.

To avoid the drawbacks and dangers of a slow reaction, the body has at its disposal another kind of local defense system that is extremely rapid. It could even be said that it goes to work immediately. Thus there is no waiting time or delay. This defense system is the inflammatory reaction, which will be described in detail in the next chapter.

The advantage of this defense system—its rapidity—is also its weakness, though. In fact, it has the drawback, due to the force of things, of being overly general. As it cannot specifically adapt to a precise invader, it has to take a one-size-fits-all approach. It is therefore a general, nonspecific, polyvalent defense mechanism. Consequently it works with less precision. As it never adapts to the type of invader it fights, its implementation never alters.

DIFFERENCES BETWEEN THE REACTIONS		
	Immune Reaction	**Inflammatory Reaction**
Speed	Slow	Rapid
Defense	Specific	General

The inflammatory reaction is a constant process. It always implements the same defense mechanisms. In the best of cases, its rapidity permits it to neutralize or destroy the invader or at least to put a break on its expansion and to limit the initial damage it might cause. This gives the body a little additional time to prepare an immune defense system specifically adapted to the invader. Although it has its limitations, the inflammatory reaction is a very valuable defense mechanism.

CONCLUSION

Many invaders—especially germs and poisons—can threaten the very survival of the body. The inflammatory reaction is one of the means used by the body to neutralize, destroy, and eliminate these invaders.

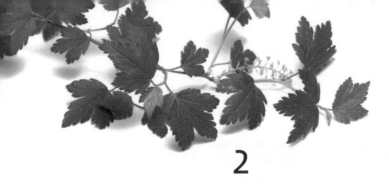

2
Physical Effects of Inflammation

Redness, Swelling, Pain, and Heat

The fundamental characteristics of the inflammation reaction were described as long ago as 30 BCE by the Roman physician Celsus. His description has been cited in reference since that time and is still applicable today. These characteristics were spelled out in Celsus's famous quadrilogy: *rubor, tumor, dolor, calor*—in other words redness, swelling, pain, heat. These are in fact the four external manifestations of an inflammatory reaction. They correspond to different processes that are taking place inside the body.

REDNESS

A human body cell cannot defend itself against an attack by germs or noxious substances on its own. This is why, when it is attacked, it sends out a distress signal, requesting aid. This signal, as we know today, primarily manifests as the release of prostaglandins by the injured cell. The immediate response to

A Little History

Celsus (Aulus Cornelius Celsus) lived during the first century BCE. This Roman citizen, physician, and author was nicknamed the Latin Hippocrates because of the volume of medical knowledge he laid out and analyzed in his book *De medicina*. He is known for his quadrilogy of the symptoms of inflammation as well as for establishing a classification of illnesses based not on their causes but on the means of healing them, to wit diet and hygiene, medications, or surgery.

this request for aid is the dilatation of the blood capillaries that irrigate the region affected by the assault.

Blood capillaries are extremely thin vessels. They are commonly described as being as fine as hair (*capillaris* is the Latin word for hair). In reality they are even finer, and they branch off as they travel into the very depths of the organs and tissues in order to irrigate them.

At the same time as the capillaries at work dilate, another phenomenon takes place. Those at rest, therefore closed, must reopen. This notion of capillaries being "closed" may be a bit surprising at first, but it can be explained as follows: If placed end to end, all the capillaries in the human body would stretch more than 62,000 miles. Together, they form an extensive irrigation network that brings blood to all of the body's deepest and most remote nooks and crannies. The surface area of the tissues this network needs to irrigate has been estimated to be more than 400 acres. As you might imagine, the quantity of blood necessary to fill the entire capillary network all at once is enormous. It so happens that the human body has only 6 to 7 quarts of blood at its disposal. This is not enough to fill all the capillaries at the same time. Hence, they are not always all filled with blood.

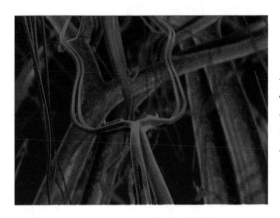

If laid end to end, all the capillaries in the human body would stretch more than 62,000 miles.

The capillary network devotes a small quantity of blood to ensuring that the entire body is minimally irrigated. The rest of the blood—in fact the bulk of it—is found in the capillaries of the regions that need it most, that is to say those that are active.

To regulate the distribution of blood, capillaries will open to attract blood to a specific region of the body, or they will close in order to expel it from that area. In this latter case, the blood is then made available to another part of the body. So some capillaries are open at certain times but closed at other times. This explains why, after we eat a large meal, we are unable to concentrate at work and feel like taking a nap. The capillaries in the brain have partially closed in order to make more blood available for the digestive organs' capillaries. If we start exercising with barbells while our food is still being digested, our digestive system will function poorly. Its capillaries will be forced to empty themselves of a considerable portion of the blood they require in order to redirect that blood to the muscles called on by the exercise.

In the event of aggression by an invader such as germs or a poison, the immediate response to the request for aid sent out by the injured cell is therefore an intensification of the circulation of blood in the endangered region. This circulatory intensification is necessary because it is the bloodstream that brings the cells what they need. The increased volume of blood encourages the nutrition and oxygenation of the cells that are fighting against the invader. It also permits quicker elimination and better expulsion of the toxic wastes and dead germs caused by these battles.

The increase in blood volume in the affected zone causes a change in the color of the skin: it reddens. Depending on the intensity of the inflammatory reaction, this red can even turn scarlet.

The inflammatory reaction caused by a bee sting, for example, causes the entire perimeter of the affected area to become red, just as the skin directly above a swollen joint will also become red. This redness is evidence of the substantial presence of blood, which itself is a sign that an inflammatory reaction has occurred.

SWELLING

The dilation of capillaries increases the porosity of their walls. Under normal circumstances these walls are permeable, allowing blood plasma (the liquid portion of blood) and various other substances to travel through the "mesh" of their membranes. But with the increase of their surface area due to dilation, the size of the "mesh" openings is increased. The walls of the capillaries therefore suddenly allow more blood plasma to enter the tissues.

The passage of blood plasma through the capillary walls is a continuous process. In fact, extracellular fluid is almost identical in composition to plasma. To simplify, we could say that extracellular fluid is blood without the red blood cells, which would also explain its whitish color. By leaving the bloodstream and traveling regularly through the tissue, the plasma permits the renewal and upkeep of the extracellular fluid. In this way the cells are continuously surrounded by a sufficient quantity of high-quality fluid.

By becoming more porous, the capillaries therefore permit greater quantities of plasma to enter the injured tissues. The plasma begins to collect in the afflicted region, and the tissues there become distended and increase in size. Celsus used the term *tumor* to designate this accumulation. Today, the preferred term is edema, tumefaction, or swelling. (A tumor is a growth due to a multiplication of cells, not an increased presence of liquid.)

The swelling that accompanies injury is a common phenomenon. The aforementioned inflamed joint will fill with fluid, and the bee sting will cause swelling of the area poisoned by the venom. Swelling will also take place following a physical shock: a sprained ankle will swell up; a blow to the head will leave a bump.

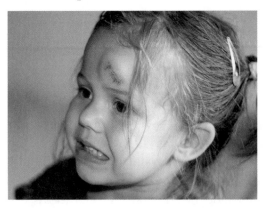

A physical shock produces swelling, better known as a bump.

The formation of the edema is the continuation and complement of the preceding effort. The body dilates the capillaries to increase the flow of blood in the area, bringing greater quantities of white blood cells, oxygen, and nutrients to the site of attack. It so happens that once the transported substances have traveled through the capillary walls, they still have to make their way to the cells. The increased quantity of extracellular fluid in the area prevents congestion of the transportation pathways. It facilitates the delivery of the transported substances to the affected cells, just as, in the opposite direction, the transport of dead cells and toxic substances to the eliminatory organs is made easier.

Furthermore, the accumulation of fluid serves a protective purpose. In the event of inflammation by toxic or poisonous substances, the irritating elements are diluted by the volume of liquid. Their potential to do damage is reduced as their concentration is diminished.

PAIN

The tissues in which the excess fluid accumulates are not infinitely expandable. The space given to the cells is limited. Consequently, the additional fluid puts pressure on them. This compresses the cells, causing a sensation of unpleasant irritation that can become outright pain. At the same time, following an attack, specialized enzymes produce substances—such as bradykinin—whose role is precisely to cause pain, which acts as an alarm signal to trigger the body's defenses.

Pain is generally considered to be a negative side effect, a useless and unpleasant symptom that we need to get rid of as soon as possible. But it has a beneficial effect that often goes unrecognized. Pain gives the body an imperative, energetic signal that it has a serious problem it needs to investigate. It triggers the mobilization of the body's defense mechanisms and the sending of "defenders" to the site of the attack. Removing the pain amounts to turning off the alarm signal. So while it is of course essential to mitigate severe pain, suppressing pain entirely can be counterproductive.

In one study a doctor who wished to test the effects of pain had a red-hot metal bar applied to both his forearms. Afterward, he immediately anesthetized one arm to curb the pain in that limb. He did not anesthetize his other arm, and that burn remained painful. However, the burn on the unanesthetized arm scarred much more quickly than the one on the

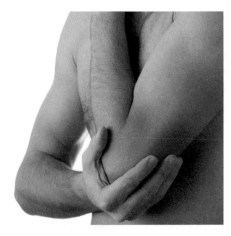

Pain encourages immobilization of the afflicted area.

anesthetized arm because the alarm signal had not been shut off.

Another beneficial effect of pain is that it encourages immobilization of the afflicted area. People instinctively put no strain on a painful area of the body in order to avoid the increased suffering that might result. Because it is not stretched or pulled by movement, the affected area is spared any additional stress.

Sometimes the inflammatory reaction induces a feeling of itchiness rather than, or in addition to, pain, for example, in cases of bee stings or sunburn. This may result when the prime cause of inflammation is attack of the tissues by the invader or from the efforts undertaken by the body to expel toxins and other irritating substances through the skin.

HEAT

The rise in temperature in the injured area is due to the intense activity taking place there. The blood circulation is strong, the combustion of toxins is elevated, the cellular exchanges are accelerated, and the elimination of wastes is increased there. In addition, different kinds of white blood cells are battling against the germs or other invaders.

All of this activity produces heat, strong enough for the afflicted individual to feel. It can sometimes even be felt by a third party who places his or her hand on the affected region, such as an inflamed joint, for example. This heat can be described as a local fever. It is beneficial, just like a fever that affects the entire body.*

Fever is certainly an expression of the defensive operations that are taking place, and thus a consequence, but it is also triggered and maintained intentionally by the body's defenses. In fact, heat stimulates cellular exchanges, blood flow, and all other physiological processes. Just as chemists in the laboratory heat the contents of their test tubes to facilitate the combination of substances that cannot be mixed at the ambient temperature, the body increases its temperature to improve its functioning. In other words, in the current context, it increases its own temperature in order to better defend itself.

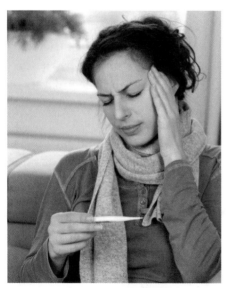

Fever comes into play to defend the body.

---

*See my book *The Healing Power of Fever: Your Body's Natural Defense against Disease* (Rochester, Vt.: Healing Arts Press, 2012).

✍

In addition to the defense processes connected with the quadrilogy drawn up by Celsus, there are other processes that occur during an inflammatory reaction.

CLEANSING

An inflammatory reaction is a battle that produces numerous corpses and wastes. It is imperative that these substances be eliminated so that they do not become a burden on the tissues, which would reduce the cells' ability to defend themselves.

These wastes are of varied origin. In the case of infection, the wastes are primarily the cadavers of slain germs, cells destroyed by the attacking agent, and white blood cells that have fallen in battle. Of course these corpses are all very small in size, but as they are numerous, they add up and eventually achieve a respectable mass. These wastes also include the poisons released by the white blood cells and those produced by the germs to defend themselves. In other cases of inflammation, the wastes requiring elimination are formed by the toxins or poisons that triggered the reaction and the cadavers of destroyed cells.

These various wastes form a more or less fluid mass that is called pus. This is the same pus that, for example, forms in a pimple, an abscess, or a wound. When elimination of these wastes takes place at the level of a mucous membrane, the wastes blend together with the secretions of this membrane. This would be the sticky phlegm that is expectorated from the lungs in bronchitis, or that drips from the nose during colds and sinusitis, or the stringy, gelatinous mucus and phlegm that accompanies the stools in cases of colitis. The term *catarrh* is used to designate the abundant release of these wastes by the mucous membranes.

REPARATION

At the end of the inflammatory reaction, the tissues have been rid of the wastes, poisons, and cadavers overloading them, but this does not mean they have been repaired. Over the course of the attack, the tissues suffered varying degrees of damage. Some cells are dead and need to be replaced. Others have been injured and their lesions need to be repaired. Breeches may have appeared on the walls of the blood capillaries, the mucous membranes, or the serous membranes (which are the protective envelopes around the organs).

These repairs can only be carried out by virtue of intense labor. This work is encouraged and sustained by the acceleration of the metabolisms triggered by the inflammatory reaction. In addition to the normal metabolic processes, there is, among others, the rapid production of fibrinogen to manufacture the frameworks needed by the tissues. There is also the creation of special proteins for repairing and scarring the lesions, closing wounds, producing new cells, and rebuilding the tissues.

The acceleration of blood circulation and the metabolisms is generally favorable to these restorative activities. Sometimes, so that this labor can be sustained, new blood capillaries are even constructed to improve irrigation of the injured tissue.

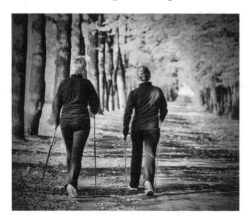

Practice of an undemanding athletic activity like walking encourages tissue repair.

Good to Know

The intensification of the metabolic processes necessary for repairing tissues can be supported, therapeutically, by the practice of a mild but sustained athletic activity, such as taking walks outside.

The intensification of physiological processes that takes place during the inflammatory reaction is therefore as favorable to restorative processes as it is to defense system processes. When everything goes well, the inflammation disappears and the assaulted tissues recover their normal state. With the cells restored, the body reassumes its normal state of balance.

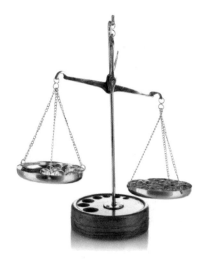

The physiological reparative processes work to restore balance in the body.

THE IMMUNE DEFENSES

What I just described is what can happen in the best of cases. There are times when the inflammatory reaction is not enough to destroy the invader, and it continues to attack and endanger the tissues. The body must consequently pursue its battle and is forced to do so with more powerful means. This invader can be a germ, a chemical or physical invader, or toxin. In order to simplify, I will go on with my explanation by talking only about what happens in the case of an invading germ.

In the previous cases, the white blood cells in play were nonspecific; in other words they were not specialized for the destruction of a specific germ but targeted all microbes. At this stage the white blood cells were neutrophils and macrophages.

- **Neutrophils** are always present in the bloodstream. They are able to enter the tissues thanks to the porosity attained by the blood capillaries in the afflicted area of the body. When they come into contact with germs at the site of infection, they release toxic substances that will destroy them.

- **Macrophages** act differently. As indicated by their name, they are larger in size (*macro*) and they swallow or eat (*phage*) their victims. Thanks to their large size, they are not satisfied with the ingestion of one or two germs but swallow hundreds at a time. These germs are then killed by the toxic substances the macrophages release to "digest" them.

If the nonspecific action of these white blood cells is not enough, specialized white blood cells—from the lymphocyte family—will be used to boost the power of the defense system. These specialized lymphocytes are designed to target a specific invader. The principle ones are the cytotoxic T cells. They kill germs by poisoning them with the help of toxic substances. Other lymphocytes known as K cells—K for killer—destroy germs with the aid of enzymes that attack the walls and organs of these microbes.

The T and K lymphocytes need to travel to the germs in order to poison or destroy them; they must come into close contact with the microbes. But other lymphocytes are capable of acting from a distance. These would be the B cells, which produce destructive substances called antibodies that are carried by the bloodstream and then the extracellular fluid to the germs.

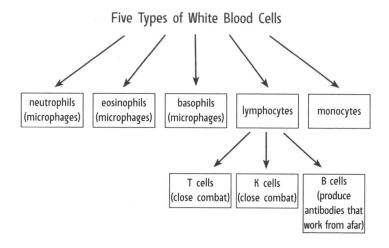

Five Types of White Blood Cells

THE MEDIATORS OF INFLAMMATION

The mobilization and coordination of all these lymphocyte "soldiers" is mediated by hundreds of substances produced by attacked cells and the various kinds of white blood cells involved in their defense. As the inflammatory reaction develops, these mediators of inflammation act on the surviving cells, which in turn act on others, in a cascading chain reaction.

There are just as many accelerating mediators as there are those that act as a brake on the inflammation. The pro-inflammatory mediators trigger, maintain, and propagate the defense system's inflammatory reactions, while the anti-inflammatory mediators curb and halt the inflammatory reactions when they have achieved their goal. The activities of these two kinds of mediators need to be effected harmoniously in order for a return to health to be possible.

It can happen that the collaboration among the inflammation mediators does not occur properly. Sometimes the production of anti-inflammatory mediators is not launched or is too weak. The action of the pro-inflammatory mediators will thus go uncurbed. The inflammation continues, eventually surpassing the goal for which it was triggered. In fact, the aggressive means by which the inflammatory reaction destroys germs or poisons also attack the tissues. Cells die and are not replaced, while others are under constant attack. The result is irritation and destruction of the tissues not by the germs and poisons alone, but partially by the defensive mechanisms themselves.

CONCLUSION

When an inflammation persists for too long a time, it will outlive its purpose. The aggressive means it uses to destroy germs or poisons also destroy the body's healthy cells. The inflammation goes from beneficial to harmful. Anti-inflammatory agents can be turned to as a remedy for this situation.

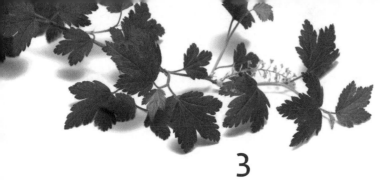

3

Fifty Illnesses Characterized by Inflammation

Common Examples of Inflammation Symptoms

We will now review the various illnesses that are characterized by inflammation. This is not an exhaustive list, however. In fact, the true number of these illnesses is quite high, as any organ or tissue can be compelled to produce an inflammatory reaction to protect itself against attack.

We will therefore discuss only the most common examples. Each review will describe the illness and outline how the typical symptoms of inflammation—redness, swelling, pain, and heat—manifest. It will also point out whether the inflammation is caused by toxic substances or an infection. The illnesses here are grouped according to the part of the body (the mouth or joints, for example) or the physiological system (the digestive or respiratory system, for example) they affect.

The illnesses characterized by inflammation generally end in the suffix *-itis,* such as otitis, rhinitis, cystitis, and so on. But a small number of diseases are an exception to this rule, although they are also inflammatory—for example, hay fever and Quincke's edema (also known as angioedema).

Inflammation can target more or less extensive areas of the body. In the case of an insect sting, it is quite small. The area is moderately large in the case of bronchitis and quite extensive in the case of hives. The inflammatory reaction can be either acute or chronic.

An inflammatory disease that is not treated properly can have serious consequences. The ones I describe here all illustrate my argument, but this does not mean that they can all be treated by the patient without the help of a medical professional.

Infection vs. Toxicity

While all infectious diseases create an inflammation of the infected area, not all inflammations are due to infections. They can also be caused by toxic substances of chemical, plant, or animal origin. Even substances that are not toxic can have an irritating effect on the tissues when present in too high a concentration. The toxins produced by the body, such as many acids (uric, pyruvic, and so on) can be included in this group. The influence of toxins in inflammations is often underestimated. But their presence in excess has a basic aggressive inflammatory effect on the tissues, which can combine with and exacerbate the harmful effect of exogenous invaders such as germs or poisons.

THE EYE AND ITS ILLNESSES

Conjunctivitis

The conjunctiva is the smooth, transparent mucous membrane that covers the outer surface of the eyeball and the inner surface of the eyelids. Inflammation of the conjunctiva is most often

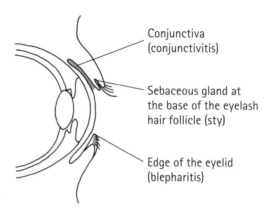

Conjunctiva
(conjunctivitis)

Sebaceous gland at
the base of the eyelash
hair follicle (sty)

Edge of the eyelid
(blepharitis)

caused by irritating substances, such as dust, tobacco smoke, and allergens (for those with allergies). It is sometimes caused by bacilli. In this event it is contagious, which is not otherwise the case.

The most visible symptom of this inflammation is the red color assumed by the white of the eye and the eyelids. Furthermore, the eyelids become swollen and the eyes become weepy. The purpose of this increased production of tears is to dilute the irritants that caused the inflammation. Pain manifests in the eyeball or by stinging and itching in the eyelids.

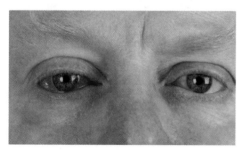

Reddening of the white part of the eye is symptomatic of conjunctivitis.

Blepharitis

This inflammation occurs on the edge of the eyelid at the location of the eyelashes. Its symptoms are similar to those of conjunctivitis.

Sty

A sty is an extremely small inflammation caused by an infection of a sebaceous gland of the eye, at the base of an eyelash follicle. Though small in size, it is located in a spot that has an abundance of nerve endings, so any inflammation here is clearly felt by a smarting sensation and stinging. The area becomes red and swollen, looking somewhat like a pimple, and releases pus.

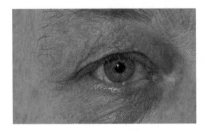

A sty is an extremely small inflammation.

THE EAR AND ITS DISEASES

Otitis

This inflammation is caused by infection (germs) or irritation (earphones, as an example). In external otitis it affects the ear canal and the eardrum; in internal otitis it affects the tympanic cavity, or middle ear. In both cases the mucous membranes in the ear turn red and become swollen with an accumulation of

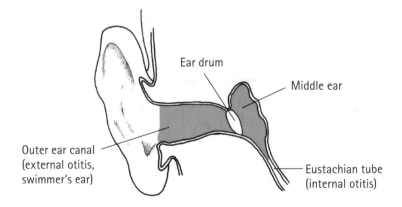

Ear drum

Middle ear

Outer ear canal
(external otitis,
swimmer's ear)

Eustachian tube
(internal otitis)

fluid and pus. The pain caused by otitis is violent, and it can cause fevers as high as 103°F.

Be advised that otitis should be treated by a trained medical professional.

THE MOUTH AND ITS DISEASES

Dental Cavity with Toothache

A cavity is a hole that forms in a tooth. This hole grows from the outside in and from the surface toward the depths. A cavity can vary in depth. If it affects only the surface of the tooth, in other words the hard protective enamel, it is not painful because there are no nerves in the enamel. When it reaches the inner layers—the dentin and the pulp—it becomes painful, as numerous sensitive nerve endings cross through these parts of the tooth.

Toothache is a sign of inflammation in the dentin and pulp, or the inner flesh of the tooth. The capillaries that irrigate this region dilate, which brings in more blood and fluid. The space in which the resulting edema forms is small, being restricted by the hard part of the tooth. The congested state that results quickly becomes quite painful, as it not only irritates the highly sensitive nerves in this space but also constricts them.

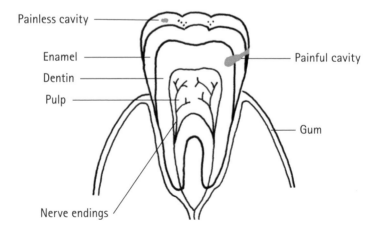

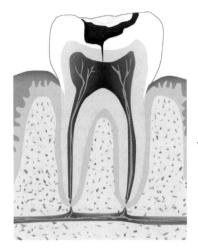

A cavity is a hole that forms in a tooth.

Some dental cavities are caused by the fermentation or putre-faction of food particles trapped between the teeth. Others are caused by the acids in foods; acids attack the teeth by leaching minerals from them. Their combined presence provides a perfect environment for the multiplication of germs, which will also attack the tooth enamel.

Gingivitis

Gingivitis is an inflammation of the gums. Gums are more specifically the mucous membranes that closely adhere to the lower portion of the teeth and cover the bone to which the teeth are fixed. The most common cause of gingivitis is dental plaque. Plaque forms naturally as a reaction between food and saliva in the mouth. Usually it is removed by brushing the teeth. If that is not the case, plaque (and also sometimes small particles of rotting food) produces germs that infect the gums and lead to inflammation. Beside these internal germs, there are others that can enter the mouth through contact with an infected object, such as food or a drinking glass. These exogenous germs will establish themselves on the gums and multiply there. In this case the inflammation will manifest not only with swelling and reddening of the gums and associated pain, but also with the formation of tiny yellow ulcers across the entirety of the gums.

Periodontitis

Periodontitis is an aggravated inflammatory state that can result from untreated gingivitis. The attack by germs is not confined to the surface of the gum but infiltrates into the area between the teeth and the gums. The gums no longer adhere directly to the teeth but become hollow and pull away, and therefore the teeth become loose. The deterioration of the gums is accompanied by inflammation, with redness, swelling, and pain. Pus forms between the teeth and the gums.

Glossitis

When the inflammation affects the tongue rather than the gums, it is known as glossitis. It is caused by infection. The tongue becomes quite red and swollen; it is accompanied by painful burning sensations.

Stomatitis

When the inflammation affects the entire mouth, it is called stomatitis. Its symptoms combine those of gingivitis and glossitis.

Canker Sores

Viruses are responsible for canker sores. They start with the formation of fluid-filled vesicles, which eventually pop and then become painful ulcers surrounded by a red halo. They can appear on the gums, tongue, and inner surface of the lips.

THE DIGESTIVE TUBE AND ITS ILLNESSES

Gastritis

Gastritis is an inflammation of the stomach. Because digestive juices are extremely acidic (having a pH of 2), they are quite irri-

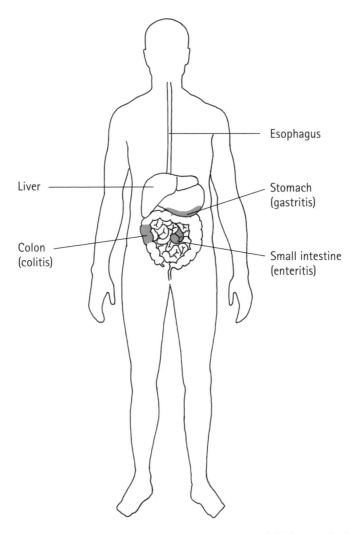

Esophagus

Liver

Stomach
(gastritis)

Colon
(colitis)

Small intestine
(enteritis)

tating. Their acidity does not normally cause any problem for the gastric mucous membrane, though, because it secretes a protective mucus that prevents the acids from coming into direct contact with it.

If inflammation is triggered in the stomach region, it may be because this layer of mucus has become too weak. This is the case with people who are often anxious or stressed. Excessive consumption of strong foods—alcohol, coffee, tea, orange juice, spices—can also contribute. Overeating or not chewing your food thoroughly is also a culprit. Stomach inflammation can also be caused by taking too much aspirin or other medications. It does sometimes have a microbial origin; most often the germ assault is attributable to *Helicobacter pylori,* bacteria whose target origin is the stomach.

The symptoms of gastric inflammation, such as redness and swelling, are not visible externally but can only be seen through a gastroscopy. The pain, on the other hand, can be felt all too clearly.

Hepatitis

This inflammation of the liver is caused by a viral infection; it is designated by the letters A, B, or C depending on which virus is responsible. The yellow tint that the patient takes on is due to bilirubin, a yellow pigment present in bile. When it is infected, the liver becomes congested with blood. The swelling of the organ that results reduces the capabilities of the bile duct. The normal transit of bile is disrupted and it stagnates. The bilirubin leaves the biliary canals and spreads into the bloodstream. It can be seen in the skin and in the whites of the eyes, which become yellow.

⚠ Caution!

Hepatitis is a serious medical condition that requires treatment by a physician.

Cholecystitis

This ailment is an inflammation of the gallbladder, the small pouch that harvests and concentrates the bile produced by the liver for the purpose of releasing it in large quantities when fatty foods are consumed. The irritation of the mucous membranes of the gallbladder is triggered by the presence of gallstones. This causes swelling of the mucous membranes, which in turn reduces the bile's ability to leave the gallbladder. It will then stagnate and rot, transforming eventually into pus. The patient becomes extremely sensitive to pressures applied to the area of this organ and to the consumption of fatty foods. It will result in sensations of pain.

Enteritis

The small intestine is a tube several yards in length that issues from the stomach. Inflammation of its walls can be caused by a microbial infection or by the poisons contained in rotten foods (shellfish, eggs, and so on). Pain is the most apparent symptom of this inflammation; it can be severe enough to force the patient to bend over. The mucous membranes of the intestine become congested. They then release more mucus than is normal, which contributes to the liquefaction of the stools (diarrhea). Any food that is eaten and comes into contact with these inflamed walls feels as if it touches an open wound. This irritation causes spasms and cramps.

Gastroenteritis

This inflammation affects the stomach and the small intestine simultaneously. It is characterized by pains and cramps. The hypersecretion of mucus leads to diarrhea. The patient may also vomit. This inflammation, more commonly known as "stomach flu," is caused by a virus.

Colitis

The colon is the final part of the digestive tube. It measures anywhere from 1½ to 2 yards in length. The mucous membranes of the colon can become inflamed due to infection or to prolonged contact with toxic substances. Such substances often come from

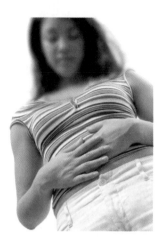

Inflammation of the mucous membranes of the colon causes colitis.

putrefaction of an alimentary bolus (the mass of food passing through the gastrointestinal tract).

In colitis the mucous membranes of the colon swell and turn red. Mucus is secreted in excessive amounts as protection against the attack. That mucus can be seen in the stools, which become quite liquid (like diarrhea). The pain can vary in intensity, depending on the case.

Appendicitis

The appendix is a small tube, about the size of a finger, that is sealed at one end and attached at its open end to the cul-de-sac of the cecum, the part of the colon that connects directly with the small intestine. Its location is therefore in the lower right-hand part of the abdomen.

Inflammation here is the result of obstruction of the appendix and the ulceration of its mucous membranes. The blockage can be caused by food waste or irritating substances that cause swelling. Although not of infectious origin, appendicitis can lead to a serious infection. The appendix and the surrounding area swell and become extremely sensitive to pressure. The pain is sharp.

If not treated, appendicitis can lead to a perforation in the walls of the appendix. The infection can then travel through

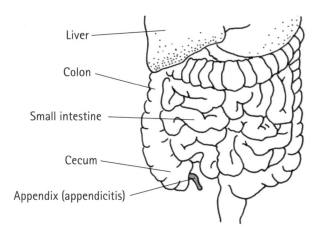

this breech and spread to the peritoneum, which is the envelope that holds all the digestive organs (peritonitis).

⚠ Caution!

If you suspect that you have appendicitis, it is urgent that you contact a physician.

Diverticulitis

The pressure exerted by stools on the walls of the lower part of the colon can sometimes be too strong, as is the case with constipation. Under the effect of this pressure, a weaker area of the walls

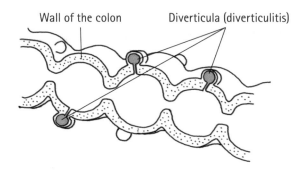

can herniate, allowing a tiny pocket or pouch of the intestinal lining, called a diverticulum, to jut out. A diverticulum can communicate with the colon, but the exchanges do not always occur properly or well. Some food particles may be able to enter yet not leave. The contents can stagnate, become infected, and attack the walls of the diverticulum. The result is an inflammation that causes severe pain in the lower belly.

THE UPPER RESPIRATORY TRACT AND ITS DISEASES

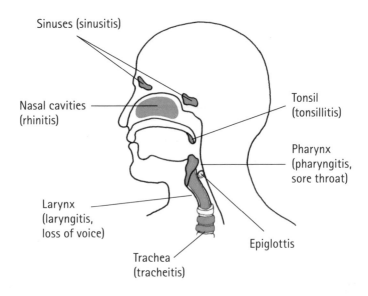

Sinuses (sinusitis)

Nasal cavities (rhinitis)

Tonsil (tonsillitis)

Pharynx (pharyngitis, sore throat)

Larynx (laryngitis, loss of voice)

Epiglottis

Trachea (tracheitis)

Sinusitis

The sinuses are cavities located in the bones of the cheeks and forehead. As hollow structures they reduce the weight of the skull and serve as resonators for the voice. The sinuses are connected to the nasal cavities by narrow passageways. Air can travel through them easily, but so can the germs responsible for infections of the nasal cavities. When those germs move into the sinuses, they extend the infection to these structures and create inflammation. Attacks of sinusitis are not uniquely caused by infection. Wastes and toxins can also collect in the sinuses and irritate the mucous membranes that line them. These wastes and germs generally come from the nasal cavities when they are over-loaded with them.

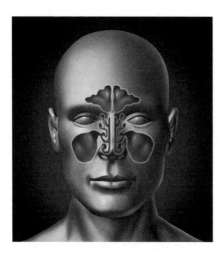

Frontal and maxillary sinuses

The attack on the mucous membranes by germs and toxins is therefore the basic cause of sinus inflammation. Obviously the red color the sinuses take on when inflamed cannot be seen. On the other hand, their swollen state is readily displayed by a feeling of congestion in the sinuses. The tubes also become swollen, which shrinks their diameter. Thus the pus generated by the dead germs and toxic substances cannot flow easily toward the nasal cavities. It stagnates and contributes to the chronic nature of this disorder.

The pain caused by this inflammation manifests in headaches and stabbing pains that increase in intensity when shaking or lowering your head. Acute attacks of sinusitis are often accompanied by fever—in other words heat.

Colds (Rhinitis or Coryza)

The infection and inflammation of the nasal cavities form strictly speaking a rhinitis, but the term *cold* is much more common.

The nasal cavities, which extend from the nostrils to the back of the oral cavity, are covered with a sticky mucous membrane that traps particles of dust, but also the germs that are transported by the inhaled air. When they get established and begin to multiply, these germs will attack the nasal mucous membranes.

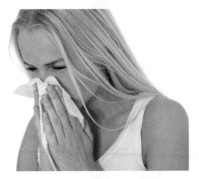

A cold: first a stuffy nose, then a runny nose

The infection causes swelling of the mucous membranes, which reduces the flow of air and makes breathing difficult. The nose has become "stuffed up" because it is congested, but this state does not last. With the inflammation fluid accumulates in the tissues. When the lesions that the virus makes in the mucous membranes become large enough, this fluid will begin to flow out. Combining with this fluid will be all the mucus secreted by glands that specialize in reaction to this attack and infection.

? Did You Know?

The French word for cold comes from a Greek word meaning "flow." It perfectly describes what takes place during a cold, because after you have caught one, your nose starts running. Another word for cold, *catarrh*, means "heavy flow."

During a cold there are no symptomatic pains, properly speaking. Burning sensations may be felt in the nose, and they can sometimes be strong. With the inflow of blood, the nose becomes red.

Sore Throat (Pharyngitis)

The pharynx is a tube that begins at the back of the nasal cavities and oral cavity. It allows the air that is inhaled to descend to the lungs and the food that is ingested to reach the esophagus. It could be described as a crossroads of digestive and respiratory tubes.

The pharynx is what is commonly called the throat. Inflammation of this organ is designated by the medical term pharyngitis. But in everyday speech it is called a sore throat. Its cause is primarily infectious.

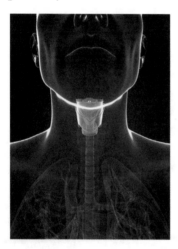

The pharynx is better known as the throat.

Inflammation of the pharynx imparts a red color to its mucous membranes. This characteristic symptom is key in diagnosing an infection of this organ. This is why a patient is asked to open his or her mouth wide and say "ah"; it makes it possible for the doctor to see the depths of the mouth. The patient can also detect this redness with the help of a mirror.

With inflammation and the accumulation of fluid in the tissues, the throat will become swollen, which makes swallowing difficult and painful. This difficulty is highlighted by the Latin word *angina,* another medical term for a sore throat, which means "to strangle, to clutch the throat." Furthermore, the patient can feel a tickling sensation at the bottom of the throat or have a hoarse voice. The heat produced by the inflammation manifests locally as well as generally in the form of fever.

⚠ Caution!

Sore throat caused by streptococcus or staphylococcus bacteria is dangerous. It can cause a very high, long-lasting fever. In this case it is imperative to consult a physician.

Rhinopharyngitis

The inflammation extends from the nose into the pharynx.

Hay Fever

See the discussion of allergies (page 70).

Tonsillitis

The tonsils are small glands formed from lymphatic tissue. They serve as part of the body's defenses against infections coming from the mouth and nose. In fact, the tonsils are placed at the crossroads of these two entryways into the body, where the larynx intersects with the back of the mouth. By opening your mouth wide, you can see them on the right and left, in the back of the throat.

The tonsils are called upon heavily during childhood, so they become infected and inflamed most often in children. During infection the tonsils become swollen and make breathing difficult. The child breathes more through the mouth than through the nose and will have a tendency to leave his or her mouth open. The tonsils will redden, and yellowish deposits of pus might be visible. Pains in the throat and ears may also accompany these symptoms.

As the tonsils are a kind of lymphatic ganglion, their role is also to filter out excess toxins. If the load of toxins is extremely heavy, these glands will labor more intensely, which will cause them to swell.

Laryngitis (Loss of Voice)

The larynx is a tube located between the pharynx and the trachea. This is the area where the vocal cords are found. The larynx is consequently the essential organ for phonation (or vocalization). In the event that it is infected by germs, has been overworked, or has been in contact with irritants like tobacco smoke or alcohol, the larynx will become inflamed. Its symptoms are similar to those of the other illnesses of the upper respiratory tract: redness, swelling that makes swallowing difficult, pain, and sometimes fever. However, these are also accompanied by a weakening of the vocal cords, which leads to hoarseness and loss of voice.

Tracheitis

The trachea is a continuation of the tube of the larynx. It conducts air into the bronchia. If infected, it becomes inflamed and painful.

THE LOWER RESPIRATORY TRACT AND ITS DISEASES

Bronchitis

At the inner end of the trachea, the tube carrying air to the lungs divides into two branches: the bronchi. They each divide into five secondary bronchi and then into fifty to eighty smaller

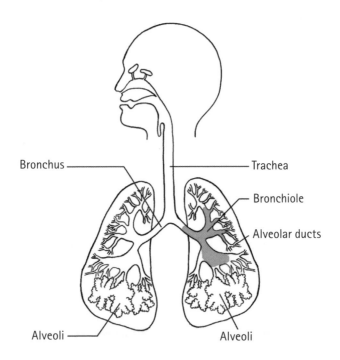

bronchioles. These latter terminate in the alveoli, where oxygen travels into the bloodstream and carbon dioxide comes into the lungs. The bronchi and bronchioles resemble the limbs of a tree that keep splitting into smaller and smaller branches. The alveoli at their tips would correspond to leaves.

Inflammation of the bronchi and bronchioles, known as bronchitis, is most often due to germs that have been carried into the body by inhaled air. But bronchitis is not always of infectious origin. Sometimes the culprit is the accumulation of wastes and toxins, or recurring irritants such as dust or tobacco smoke.

At the onset of bronchial inflammation, the accumulation of tissues that have been destroyed by the germs and germ corpses leads to the formation of pus. Added to the pus is the mucus secreted by the glands of the bronchial membranes as

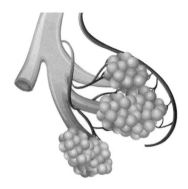

The passage of oxygen into the bloodstream and carbon dioxide into the lungs takes place in the alveoli.

defense against the microbial invasion. Together they form the phlegm that will be expectorated. Initially this phlegm is not very abundant, but it is thick. It will increase in quantity and become more fluid as the infection progresses and the inflammatory reaction develops.

The inflammation of the bronchi makes them very sensitive and painful. They are especially painful during coughing, which is the effort made by the body to rid itself of the wastes that are burdening the bronchi and bronchioles. A slight fever can also appear.

This infection can sometimes travel down to the ends of the bronchiole network and reach the alveoli. At this point the infection and inflammation will be affecting the entire lungs; this is bronchopneumonia. If it affects the envelope holding the lungs—the pleura—it is pleurisy.

⚠ **Caution!**

If you suspect that you have either bronchopneumonia or pleurisy, it is essential to get medical treatment.

Asthma

See the discussion of asthma on page 71.

THE BLOOD VESSELS AND THEIR DISEASES

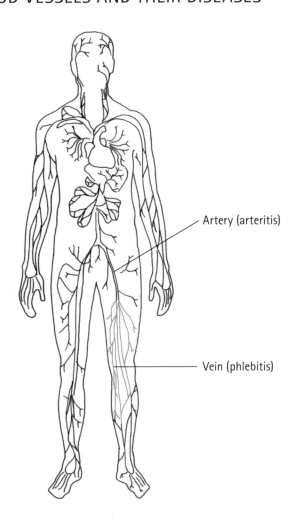

Artery (arteritis)

Vein (phlebitis)

Phlebitis

In order to circulate easily, the blood requires a certain level of fluidity, and the vessels through which it travels must be clear of any deposits. If the blood is thickened by the toxins it is transporting, it will circulate more slowly in vessels. If the situation develops—particularly if those vessels have been reduced in diameter by deposits—circulation can slow to the point that the blood coagulates, forming deposits that partially clog the vein. The vein is attacked by the stagnant blood and becomes inflamed.

Inflammation of the veins, known as phlebitis, occurs most frequently in the legs. This is where the venous blood has the greatest difficulty circulating because it has to overcome the force of gravity to ascend back toward the heart.

A case of phlebitis in a leg manifests in sharp localized pain and pain in the groin above the afflicted limb. If the vein is visible, the red color it has assumed can be seen. Edema will form at the ankle.

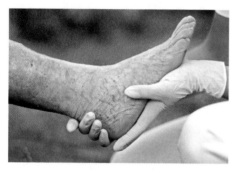

Poor venous circulation is evident in varicose veins.

Arteritis

Artery inflammation also afflicts the lower limbs most often. Its causes and symptoms are the same as those of phlebitis.

Hemorrhoids

Hemorrhoids are varicose veins (veins that are abnormally swollen) in the rectum and anus. They can be present without causing the slightest inflammation. However, because of the swelling of the veins and the twisting course they take, the circulation of blood is slowed, and any irritants transported by the blood will remain in contact longer with the walls of the vessels. This can cause an inflamed state with additional swelling and pain.

THE KIDNEYS AND BLADDER
AND THEIR DISEASES

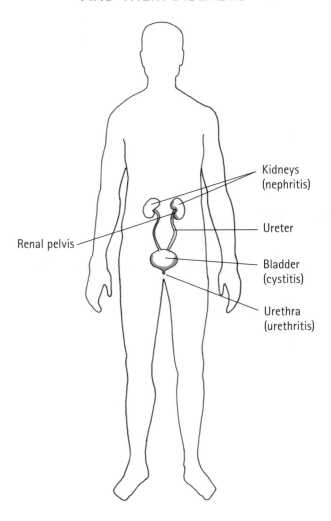

Kidneys
(nephritis)

Ureter

Renal pelvis

Bladder
(cystitis)

Urethra
(urethritis)

Nephritis

Germs are responsible for infection and inflammation of the kidneys. The term *nephritis,* meaning kidney inflammation, is rarely used by itself, however; it is generally accompanied by a prefix that defines the exact area of the kidney that is afflicted. For example, glomerulonephritis is the term used to describe inflammation of the renal glomeruli (filtration units), interstitial nephritis describes inflammation of the medulla interstitium (the tissue surrounding the tubules that carry fluid through the kidney), and pyelonephritis describes inflammation of the pyelum (or renal pelvis, where urine collects before being passed to the bladder).

The germs responsible for the inflammation come from an infected organ elsewhere in the body. For example, they may come from the bladder during an attack of cystitis or from the throat during a case of pharyngitis.

When they become inflamed, the mucous membranes of the kidneys become swollen, which reduces the diameter of or even blocks the channels responsible for urine flow. This is accompanied by lumbar pain.

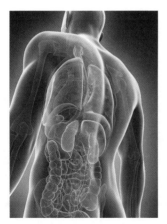

The kidneys are situated in the middle of the back, hidden under the last ribs.

⚠ Caution!

Kidney inflammation can have serious consequences. Consultation with a trained medical professional is a priority.

Cystitis

This is inflammation of the mucous membranes that line the inside of the bladder. It is generally accompanied by inflammation of the ureter.

Infection is the primary cause of cystitis. Germs attach themselves to the walls of the bladder and begin to multiply. They and the toxins they secrete assail the mucous membranes. The membranes become red and irritated. They become overly sensitive to the pressure exerted on them by urine collecting in the bladder, so that even a small quantity of urine results in the desire to urinate. Burning sensations and pain appear in the lower belly and increase severely during urination. The entire pelvic region becomes congested. Fever sometimes accompanies this infection.

⚠ Caution!

Cystitis that lasts longer than three days should be treated by a physician.

🖐 Good to Know

Some attacks of cystitis are due not to infection but to an extremely acidic terrain. High concentrations of acids in the urine can make it extremely irritating. This can result in a painful inflammation of the bladder, accompanied by burning sensations, without any fever.

Urethritis

The urethra is the tube through which urine passes from the bladder on its way out of the body. When it is inflamed, which is most often caused by an infection, its end becomes red, and it becomes congested and expels pus. Often urethritis is accompanied by a mild fever.

THE JOINTS, MUSCLES, TENDONS, AND THEIR DISEASES

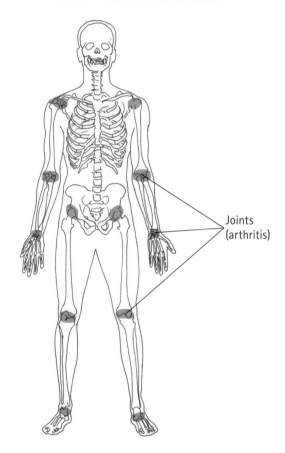

Joints
(arthritis)

Arthritis

Arthritis is the inflammation of a joint. It is often commonly referred to as rheumatism.

There are a number of different kinds of arthritis or rheumatism, depending on the joint that is affected and how greatly it is afflicted. Basically, though, the inflammation manifests in a similar fashion in all joints. The causes of this inflammation are the presence of toxins, and more specifically, acids.

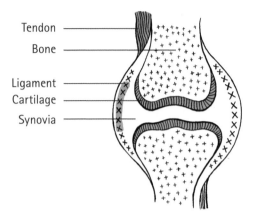

Tendon

Bone

Ligament

Cartilage

Synovia

The swelling of an inflamed joint is visible externally. The joint, for example the knee, increases in size because of the accumulation of fluid in the surrounding tissues. An excess amount of fluid also accumulates in the intra-articular space, or synovial envelope. The skin directly over the afflicted joint becomes red and hot to the touch. The increased sensitivity of the different parts of the joint—the bone surfaces in contact with each other, the ligaments, the synovial envelope, and so forth—causes pain that can be either constant or stimulated only by movement.

? Did You Know?

The word *rheumatism*, which is interchangeable with *arthritis*, comes from the Greek *rheuma*, which means "flux" or "flow," in reference to the accumulation of fluid.

Stiff Neck and Lumbago

The inflammations involved here are those of the muscles and not the joints: the neck muscles for a stiff neck and those of the lower back for lumbago. They most often develop in those individuals with an acidic terrain.

The concentration of acids in the cellular fluids that irrigate the muscles are a constant source of irritation. If the acid level rises, as it might following intense or protracted physical effort, inflammation can erupt. A sudden movement, holding the neck or back in an unusual position for any length of time, or even prolonged contact with something cold can also trigger this condition.

In cases of stiff neck and lumbago, the muscles are congested and subject to spasm. Intense pain manifests with every movement.

Tendinitis

The muscles are connected to the bones by the cordlike tendons. Following sustained physical effort, which causes the production of acidic toxins, a tendon can become inflamed. This is all the more likely when the terrain is already acidic. For example, playing tennis places great demand on the elbow. This can result in inflammation of the tendons in this joint, a condition commonly described as "tennis elbow."

But tendinitis can also occur in other joints, such as the wrists and ankles, if excessive physical activity has overworked them (too much use of clippers or pruners, walking in the sand, too much use of a computer mouse, and so on).

The inflamed tendon becomes quite painful and prevents

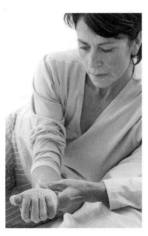

Tendinitis often manifests in the wrists of those who spend a lot of time working on a computer.

movement of the affected region. This area can become red and somewhat swollen.

Gout

Gout is a sudden and violent inflammation. Most often it affects the joint of the big toe. It is caused by a strong concentration of uric acid in the joint. The toe becomes extremely painful. The patient cannot stand even the weight of a blanket on it. The toe becomes clearly swollen and red. It is sometimes accompanied by fever.

Neuritis

Nerves that have been weakened by irritating substances (such as germs, acids, or toxins) or by trauma (such as a blow or contact with a cold surface) can become inflamed. The inflamed zone becomes sensitive, painful, and slightly congested, and sometimes it turns red. Neuritis commonly occurs in an optic nerve, facial nerve, intercostal nerve, or nerve of the ear.

Sciatica

Inflammation of the sciatic nerve is often caused by pinching of some portion of the nerve, usually in the lumbar spine. The pain

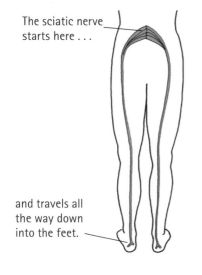

The sciatic nerve starts here . . .

and travels all the way down into the feet.

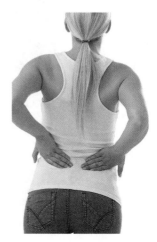

Sciatic pain can be quite fierce.

this causes is quite sharp. It begins in the buttocks and travels down the leg, sometimes all the way into the foot. The pain follows, in fact, the trajectory of the sciatic nerve. An acidic terrain that is loaded with toxins will increase the irritation of this nerve. Freedom of movement is restricted.

THE SKIN AND ITS DISEASES

Acne

The sebaceous glands release sebum, which can sometimes oxidize at the exit of the gland and harden. The result is a blackhead that prevents the flow of sebum to the outside. The trapped sebum and the dying cells that accumulate there trigger an infection. This inflames the gland and the surrounding area, which become swollen. The result of this is a large, pus-filled, red pimple that is warm and sometimes painful.

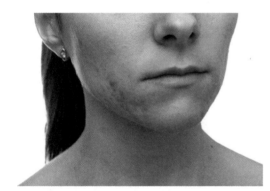

When sebum can no longer flow freely and infection prevails, the result is acne.

Eczema

Eczema occurs when the skin is in contact with irritating substances of internal origin (such as acids and toxins) that it eliminates in perspiration or of external origin (such as chemical products). The skin can then become inflamed. Red patches develop as a result of the inflow of blood to the region. The zone

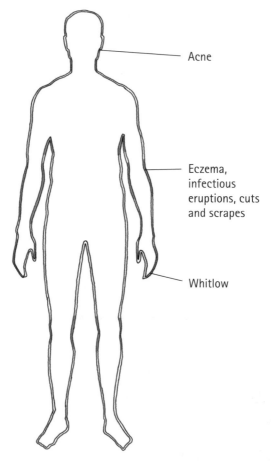

Acne

Eczema, infectious eruptions, cuts and scrapes

Whitlow

of patches is more swollen than the rest of the body. It is speckled with small blisters filled with a thick liquid. When it seeps out, it dries on contact with the air and forms a crust. The skin feels itchy and is hot to the touch.

👆 **Good to Know**

The majority of eczema cases have not an external cause but an internal one: an excess of acid toxins that the body is trying to get rid of by expelling them through sweat.

Infectious Eruptions

Some infectious diseases, like the childhood illnesses of measles, rubella, chicken pox, scarlet fever, and so forth, cause skin eruptions that are one of their characteristic symptoms. The skin becomes inflamed because its glands are expelling numerous toxic and irritating substances: dead cells, germ cadavers, microbial toxins, and metabolic wastes. The eruptions are red, swollen, hot, and itchy.

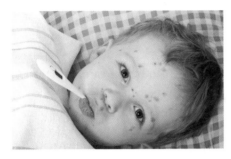

This skin eruption is a characteristic sign of measles.

Insect Stings

The venom that accompanies the stings of bees, wasps, and other insects (as well as the germs they can deposit at the site of the sting) attacks the skin. The resulting irritation triggers an inflammation of the afflicted area. It swells up to form a pimple or edema. The zone is red, painful, hot, and itchy.

Superficial Cuts

Small superficial wounds (cuts and scrapes) become inflamed because of the damage they cause to the skin. The cut or scrape may become swollen, red, and sensitive. If germs enter the wound, the infection will lead to the formation of pus.

Whitlow

This is an infection of the fingertip. The infection begins when germs come into contact with broken or injured skin at the tip of the finger. The resulting inflammation makes the finger red, swollen, hot, and extremely painful.

ALLERGIES AND ASTHMA

Hay Fever and Other Allergies

Unlike the common cold that rages in winter, hay fever is allergenic in origin, not infectious. As its name indicates, hay fever is caused by irritating substances given off by plants, more specifically the pollen of certain flowers, grasses, herbs, and even trees. When this pollen comes into contact with the nasal mucous membranes of allergic individuals, it triggers a strong inflammatory reaction in the nose region that often extends to the eyes.

The reddening of the mucous membranes can be seen primarily around the eyes; the eyelids assume this characteristic color of inflammation. The swelling affects all the mucous membranes in the area, as well as the eyes. The accumulation of fluid in the tissues leads to an abnormally high release of fluids. The nose runs liberally, and the eyes weep copiously. The affected parts of the face grow hot. The inflammatory reaction is not painful, but it causes intense itching sensations that make sufferers sneeze violently and repeatedly or rub their eyes.

The same reactions are possible with other allergens, like dust or animal dander.

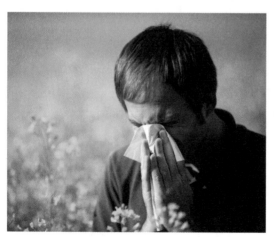

Inflammation is triggered when pollen comes into contact with the nasal mucous membranes of an allergic individual.

Asthma

In asthma the inflammatory reaction manifests in the region of the bronchi. They can become inflamed due to exposure to environmental irritants, allergens, or an accumulation of toxins. The inflammatory reaction reduces the capacity of the bronchial network in a host of ways. To begin the blood capillaries located in the walls of the bronchi increase in diameter to accommodate greater blood flow. Thus they take up more space than they do normally, which consequently constricts the space for the bronchi. The bronchial mucous membranes hypersecrete mucus as a measure of protection against the irritant causing the inflammation, but this only shrinks the space available for breathing even more. This congestion and constriction are further complicated by spasms of the muscles responsible for the dilation and constriction of the bronchi.

The result is that patients often have great difficulty inhaling enough air into their lungs and experience an asthma attack. They may feel like they are suffocating. Their difficulty in getting enough oxygen can cause panic, and the phases of suffocation may culminate in strong coughing attacks.

Hives

Hives is an allergic inflammatory reaction during which the skin becomes covered by patches of swollen pink wheals or welts, similar to those caused by nettle sting. These wheals are prominent and form the headquarters of a disagreeably burning, itching sensation. They disappear after several hours but can reappear elsewhere on the body.

Quincke's Edema

Quincke's edema, also known as angioedema, is an inflammatory reaction that is triggered in many cases by allergies. Like hives, it causes swelling, but in this case the swelling occurs in deep (subcutaneous) tissue, rather than being on the surface of the skin. The portions of the body that are most commonly affected are the eyelids and face, but it can also strike the tongue, throat, and other parts of the body. In these latter cases, it poses a danger of shrinking the airways.

⚠ Caution!

If your tongue or throat appear to be swelling,
see a doctor immediately.

THE SEXUAL ORGANS AND THEIR DISEASES

Genital Mycosis (Candidiasis)

The fungi and yeasts responsible for incidences of mycosis are germs. When they colonize the mucous membranes of the male or female genital organs, they create an inflammation, as is the case with any other microbial infection.

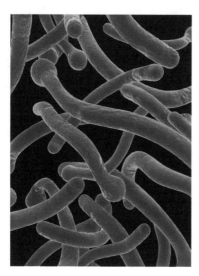

The fungus Candida albicans *is responsible for many cases of mycosis.*

One of the fungi responsible for many mycosis cases is *Candida albicans.* The mucous membranes on which it develops are assaulted by its presence and the toxins it produces. They become red and inflamed. Itching accompanies this inflammation, as does a burning sensation.

Prostatitis

The prostate is a gland located beneath the male bladder. With age it tends to become enlarged (hypertrophy), which shrinks the diameter of the urethra. This slows down the flow of urine, which can lead to infections. When this happens the prostate becomes inflamed. It becomes swollen and urination becomes difficult and painful. Fever can accompany this condition.

FEVER

To bring this overview of diseases with inflammation to a close, I need to discuss fever. Fever, as it occurs with the flu, for example, is itself an inflammatory reaction. It is not restricted to a closely confined area of the body but manifests throughout. The four major symptoms of inflammation are present. The skin of a feverish individual takes on a reddish tinge, which can easily be seen on the face and throat. The patient becomes a bit swollen, because his or her body is retaining liquid. (At the onset of a fever, the elimination of fluid via urination and perspiration drops in order to reduce the concentration of wastes in contact with the cells and to allow white blood cells to circulate more freely in the tissues. It is only after a fever spike that sweating begins.*) The body of a feverish individual aches and is quite sensitive to pain. And of course the fourth symptom of

---

*See my book *The Healing Power of Fever.*

inflammation, heat, is readily evident in the elevation of body temperature.

CONCLUSION

Inflammatory diseases are characterized by four major symptoms: redness, swelling, pain, and heat. These symptoms can take different forms depending on the organ or site of the inflammation, but they are always present.

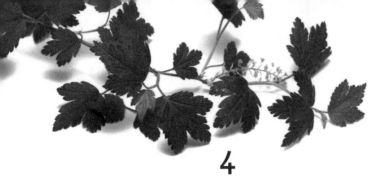

4

How Anti-Inflammatory Agents Work

The Biochemistry of Inflammation

Anti-inflammatory agents are substances capable of reducing or even eliminating the reactions of inflammation. They moderate the excessive manifestations of inflammation and ease the patient's suffering. To understand how they work, it is necessary to briefly examine the biochemistry of inflammation and to take particular notice of a fundamental mediator of this defense-system process: prostaglandins.

 Good to Know

A mediator is a substance that possesses the ability to trigger a specific reaction in the body.

THE PROSTAGLANDINS

As soon as a cell comes under attack, it releases two kinds of prostaglandins (as well as other substances that, in order to keep things simple, we will not discuss).

The first we will call the prostaglandins of war. When cells come under attack, these prostaglandins mediate (trigger) the mechanisms that dilate the blood capillaries in the area and thereby increase their permeability, which allows greater quantities of blood plasma to travel into the tissues to form an edema. They also facilitate the transmission of pain signals that inform the body's defenses of the attack.

As our name for them indicates, the prostaglandins of war prepare and trigger the body's defensive reactions. This is not a passive defense, however, insofar as white blood cells attack and fight the invader. The prostaglandins arouse, excite, and bring to a boil the attack systems with which the body strikes the enemy in order to destroy it.

Any battle will cause much damage, however. This is equally true whether it is a war between human beings (resulting in numerous dead and wounded, along with the destruction of homes, roadways, and other infrastructure) or a battle inside the body (resulting in the destruction or injury of tissues, the loss of white blood cells, and so on). Thus a battle cannot be endless. If it goes on too long, serious damage will result. A brake must be applied to the attack-and-destroy process that the body has implemented.

The responsibility for this falls to the second kind of prostaglandins, which we will call the prostaglandins of peace. Their activity consists of contracting the blood capillaries and reducing their permeability, which shrinks the edema. It also limits the transmission of pain signals.

The purpose of the prostaglandins of peace is to mitigate, calm, and even halt the inflammatory reaction. The typical activities of peacetime—construction and repair—can then take place. They correspond to convalescence and a return to health.

The prostaglandins of peace therefore stand in opposition to the prostaglandins of war. While the latter cause inflammation, the activities of the prostaglandins of peace are anti-inflammatory. These opposing modes of activity are useful for the body. They permit it to monitor and regulate the inflammatory reaction—in other words, to ensure that the defense processes persist for an appropriate length of time and are followed by repair work.

ACTION OF PROSTAGLANDINS		
	War **(Pro-Inflammatory)**	**Peace** **(Anti-Inflammatory)**
Capillaries	Dilate	Contract
Permeability	Increases	Decreases
Edema	Forms	Is reabsorbed
Transmission of Pain Signals	Facilitated	Halted

ACUTE AND CHRONIC INFLAMMATION

Normally, the production of the pro-inflammatory prostaglandins is followed some time later by that of anti-inflammatory prostaglandins. The burst of defensive activity achieves its goal and is then put to rest. Under these circumstances, the condition is described as an acute inflammation. It is characterized by the limited time frame of its duration, a limit that is imposed by a sufficient presence of prostaglandins of peace to counter the defensive efforts that are no longer serving any helpful purpose.

Sometimes, though, an imbalance is established between these two opposing forces, and it works to the benefit of the defensive processes, which continue their activities for too long a period. When the body is unable to curb these pro-inflammatory activities with anti-inflammatory prostaglandins, they exceed their bounds. The cells of the inflamed tissues can be injured and even killed. The tissues suffer lesions and harden. The pain connected to the inflammatory process persists and causes the patient to suffer for longer than is necessary. This condition is known as a chronic inflammation.

During acute inflammations, anti-inflammatory agents are used primarily to soothe the pain felt by the patient. In chronic inflammations they make it possible to protect the tissues from damage and also ease the patient's suffering.

Chronic inflammation has many possible causes. Most often it results from the fact that the body's protective forces—which depend on the anti-inflammatory prostaglandins—are too weak in comparison with those of its attack forces—which depend on the pro-inflammatory prostaglandins. It may also be that the cause of the inflammation has not been removed; in other words an infection, poison, or allergen has not yet been neutralized, and its continued presence ensures that the body's defensive reactions will continue. Another possible cause is an overload of toxins in the cellular terrain; in this case the body's defenses will mobilize against the toxins and the damage they cause, and they will remain active for as long as the toxins persist.

Whatever the cause might be, an inflammatory reaction that persists or is excessively intense will become harmful to the body. It must be curbed in order to protect the body and give it time for repair and rest. Anti-inflammatory substances are the remedies to use for this purpose.

THE CAUSES OF
CHRONIC INFLAMMATION

- Deficit of anti-inflammatory prostaglandins
- The infection causing the inflammation persists
- Poisons and allergens have not been neutralized
- Overload of toxins

Chronic Inflammation and Cancer

Chronic inflammation can, over time, lead to cancer. In a case of chronic inflammation, the body is under constant attack by both the causal agent (the germ, poison, or toxin) and, to an equal extent, the inflammatory defensive mechanisms. While this can result in the total destruction of a cell, it can also lead to mere injury. In some cases this injury will involve the cell's genetic material. Alteration of a cell's genetic material can lead to a chaotic multiplication of the cell, which can lead to the growth of a tumor. This is only possible, however, if the damaged terrain permits it and the immune system is too weak to stop it.

Preventive measures for avoiding this escalation of cellular injury and abnormal growth consist of effectively treating chronic inflammation. The means to succeed rest not only in taking anti-inflammatory agents, but also in removing or neutralizing the primary cause of the inflammation.

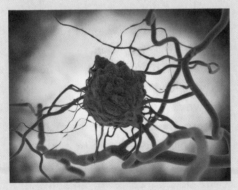

The chronic nature of inflammation can lead, over time, to cancer.

HOW ANTI-INFLAMMATORIES WORK

Given the role prostaglandins play in inflammations, there are two ways that an anti-inflammatory therapy can proceed:

1. It can aim to block the production of the pro-inflammatory prostaglandins of war (when they are in excess).
2. It can seek to increase the production of anti-inflammatory prostaglandins of peace (when they are insufficient).

ANTI-INFLAMMATORY THERAPY	
The Two Aspects	**The Two Means**
Block pro-inflammatory prostaglandins	Plants, aspirin and other pharmaceuticals, cortisone
Increase anti-inflammatory prostaglandins	Omega-3 essential fatty acids

The first of these two methods involves the use of anti-inflammatory remedies. In natural medicine these would include plants; in allopathic medicine they include aspirin, cortisone, and other pharmaceuticals. These remedies block the production of pro-inflammatory prostaglandins thanks to various substances they contain.

The consequence of their use is that the body's inflammatory reactions are thwarted. Without the continued presence of pro-inflammatory prostaglandins, the production of white blood cells is clearly restrained, if not halted outright. The capillaries are no longer dilated and edema (swelling) is reduced, which hampers the passage of white blood cells toward the affected tissues. For lack of fighters, the inflammatory reaction grinds to a halt. In this way the objective—the end of the inflammatory process—is achieved via an external supply of prostaglandin blockers, rather than the normal action of anti-inflammatory prostaglandins produced by the body.

The second measure—increasing the production of anti-inflammatory prostaglandins—relies not on medicines but on nutrition. It consists of supplying, in sufficient quantities, the essential nutrients for the production of anti-inflammatory prostaglandins, to wit, omega-3 essential fatty acids. When increased in number, these anti-inflammatory prostaglandins can counter the destructive inflammatory activities, and as a consequence the inflammation fades away.

A BRIEF HISTORY OF ANTI-INFLAMMATORIES

Since the dawn of time, human beings have used anti-inflammatory agents in the form of medicinal plants. While they did not grasp how these plants worked on the biochemical level, they were perfectly aware of their effectiveness. Two plants stand out in particular among those they used: willow and meadowsweet.

White Willow

In ancient Mesopotamia, as early as 5000 BCE, the Sumerians used willow leaves for treating various pains, which is evidence of their knowledge of this plant's anti-inflammatory properties. They inscribed the recipe for preparing the healing brew on clay tablets that have since been unearthed. An Egyptian papyrus from 1550 BCE also describes the virtues and uses of willow. The same plant was recommended for the same uses in ancient China. And Hippocrates, the father of medicine (fourth century BCE), recommended a preparation of white willow bark for fighting arthritic pain and fever.

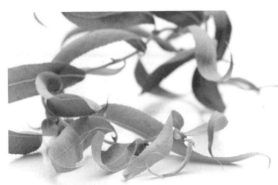

White willow

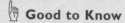

Good to Know

The ancients noted and made use of the fact that anti-inflammatories have an anti-fever effect. The two effects are in fact related. By reducing the intensity of the metabolisms that take place during the inflammatory reaction, anti-inflammatory remedies reduce the production of heat and, thus, fever. We should not forget that fever is a general inflammatory reaction.

In the first century CE, Dioscorides, a Greek botanist and physician, and author of a treatise on more than five hundred medicinal plants, prescribed willow leaves that had been macerated in wine for the treatment of lumbar pain. Galen, a physician of second-century Rome, considered then to be the greatest doctor of antiquity, also used willow; in fact, he claimed that few other medications had as many uses as this plant.

The willow is not only known in Europe and Asia but is also used on the American continent. Numerous Amerindian people made use of it; for example, some tribes of California employed it against back pain, and the Pima of Arizona used it to treat fever. Willow was used throughout the Middle Ages and into the modern era, and it remains a staple of contemporary natural medicine. Dr. Jean Valnet (1920–1995), dubbed "Doctor Nature" and the author of various books on the virtues of plants, described white willow as the "anti-pain tree," thereby clearly highlighting its anti-inflammatory properties.

Meadowsweet

The history of meadowsweet, sometimes called queen of the meadow, also stretches far back into antiquity. The Greeks and Romans were fully aware of its anti-inflammatory properties. Hippocrates discovered that this plant was effective against

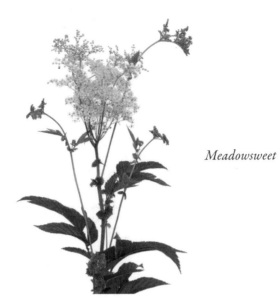

Meadowsweet

the pain of arthritis and other illnesses. His contemporary Theophrastus compiled a treatise on plants that earned him the title of "father of botany." Cognizant of meadowsweet's wonderful properties, Theophrastus grew it in his own garden. He recommended it especially for lowering fever. Dioscorides, of the first century CE, prescribed this plant for an extremely inflammatory disease: gout. And during the Middle Ages, meadowsweet was used against the skin eruptions that accompanied diseases like smallpox and measles.

In the mid-1800s meadowsweet experienced a new boom in popularity. A French priest, Father Obriot, restored its use to honor. He rightly extolled its draining and anti-inflammatory properties, which were shown to reduce pain and swelling in joints. During this time the plant was regarded as a panacea against joint pain. Intrigued by the popularity of this plant, a doctor from Lyon performed extensive research on meadowsweet and confirmed its effectiveness against arthritic inflammations.

Why is meadowsweet effective against inflammation?

Research on this subject shows that its active principle—salicylic acid—is also present in willow. But the discovery of this active principle brings us to the story of the creation of the most extensively used anti-inflammatory medication in the world—aspirin.

Aspirin

Worldwide consumption of aspirin is estimated to be some 40,000 tons a year, amounting to 120 billion 300 mg tablets. For a population of seven billion people, this works out annually to 17 tablets a person. This is an enormous figure and shows the important role played by anti-inflammatory agents in current medical treatments. These treatments could just as easily rely on natural substances that fight against inflammation.

Aspirin's history is quite interesting, as it illustrates how this remedy, like so many others, was developed from a medicinal plant.

The discovery of aspirin involves two main players from the plant world: willow and meadowsweet. As modern chemistry developed in scope and knowledge, many researchers undertook to discover why these two plants, which had been used throughout human history, were effective as anti-inflammatories.

In the eighteenth century, the principal remedy used against fevers and infections was "Peruvian bark" (cinchona), a remedy rich in quinine. But as it became rarer and more expensive, alternatives were sought. This is how in 1763 an English pastor, the Reverend Edward Stone, came to experiment with willow bark. He gave it every four hours, in powder form, to more than fifty of his patients. Because of the success of his treatment, willow bark was henceforth used regularly in the treatments of that time.

In 1829 a French pharmacist, Joseph Leroux, attempted to discover willow's active properties. He boiled powdered bark in water and then concentrated the resulting liquid as much as

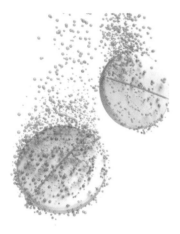

Aspirin is regarded as a universal panacea.

possible. He obtained soluble crystals that he baptized *salicyline,* inspired by the Latin word for willow, *salix.* Later researchers would purify these crystals to obtain an acid that they named salicylic acid.

In tandem with these studies of willow, other research was being performed on meadowsweet. In 1835 German researcher Karl Löwig extracted from meadowsweet an acid that he named *spirsaure* ("spiric acid," after the former Latin genus name for the plant, *Spiraea*). He subsequently discovered that this substance was chemically identical to the salicylic acid of the willow tree. In this way researchers were able to identify with greater precision the substance responsible for the anti-inflammatory effect of both plants.

Researchers found that they could prepare a remedy from natural extracts of the plants, and it was effective against pain and arthritic inflammation, but it produced very alarming side effects, chief among them burning sensations in the stomach, which if unaddressed could lead to lesions and hemorrhages. In an attempt to avoid these drawbacks, attempts to synthesize the active molecule in the laboratory were undertaken. In 1859 German chemist Adolph Kolbe succeeded in creating a chemical synthesis of salicylic acid. This substance proved to have effective

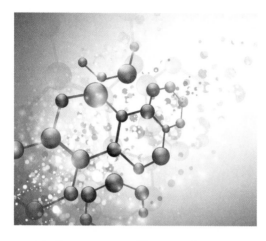

The aspirin molecule: acetylsalicyclic acid

anti-inflammatory effects and was increasingly prescribed by doctors, but like its predecessors, it was difficult for the stomach to tolerate. Research therefore continued.

Later studies led to a very similar compound that was easier to produce, more active, and—an important advantage—better tolerated by the digestive tract. This compound was acetylsalicylic acid, which today we call aspirin. The perfection of this remedy was the work of the German chemist Felix Hoffmann, who in 1897 synthesized acetylsalicylic acid from the salicylic acid of meadowsweet by acetylation. Aspirin was born.

? Did You Know?

The "a" in *aspirin* refers to the process of acetylation, while the particle "spir" refers to the so-called spiric acid of meadowsweet.

Aspirin takes effect much more quickly than natural extracts of willow and meadowsweet. Its action is also stronger. However, its effect does not last as long, and the problems of stomach lesions and irritation persist.

Purification vs. Synergism

The gastrointestinal side effects are a major obstacle to the use of aspirin and other similar remedies, but this obstacle does not exist for natural extracts of willow or meadowsweet. In fact, this is a problem that crops up repeatedly with "pure" pharmaceuticals produced from a plant or synthesized in a laboratory. These pharmaceuticals are made up solely of whatever particular compound is considered to be a plant's active constituent. But this means that the active constituent is isolated, rather than being surrounded by all the other substances found in the whole plant that work in synergy with it. These other synergistic substances are called cofactors. Their collective action ensures that the plant is easily tolerated by the body. When the cofactors are withdrawn from the primary constituent, the remedy acquires undesirable side effects, such as attacking the stomach.

In this regard it is helpful to read what French doctor and herbalist Max Tétau wrote: "The entire plant has a clearer and more complex action than one or more of its isolated active principles. It forms a natural synergic whole of a simpler and more manageable therapeutic activity."*

This is the reason why plants like willow and meadowsweet, to cite only those two, are today regaining their popularity as whole-plant remedies and natural extracts.

---

*La phytothérapie rénovée (Paris: Éditions Maloine, 1972).

Other Anti-Inflammatory Pharmaceuticals: The NSAIDs

Since the development of aspirin, many other pharmaceutical anti-inflammatories have been developed. Most can be grouped with aspirin in the category of pharmaceuticals known as non-steroidal anti-inflammatory drugs, or NSAIDs. These include the propionic acid derivatives (such as ibuprofen and naproxen), the oxicams (such as piroxicam and meloxicam), the coxibs (such as celecoxib), and so on. They are just as effective as aspirin. The big difference between the two is that aspirin inhibits the clotting of the blood for a long period of time, which is not the case with other NSAIDs.

Cortisone

Some forty years after the invention of aspirin, another powerful anti-inflammatory substance was discovered. It came not from a plant but from a substance produced by the body itself: a hormone called cortisone that is released by the adrenal glands.

In the early 1900s, knowledge of the endocrine glands was still quite sketchy. But extensive research conducted over the century led to attempts to pinpoint their exact role. In particular we can thank Argentine physiologist Bernardo Houssay (1887–1971) for identifying the role of the adrenal glands. Among other things he discovered that these glands produce secretions, which would later be called hormones, with strong physiological effects. The American chemist Edward Kendall (1886–1972) identified one of those secretions as cortisone and noted its anti-inflammatory effect, and its potential for therapeutic benefit. Four years' work was necessary to successfully synthesize it in the laboratory. At this point the substance was available for experimentation on patients.

The first trials were conducted at the end of the 1940s by American rheumatologist Philip Hench (1896–1965). His treatment of patients stricken with rheumatoid arthritis was so successful that it spawned an enormous enthusiasm for cortisone that still exists today.

The laboratory synthesis of cortisone makes it possible to manufacture medications with a high concentration of active principles. They are much more powerful than the cortisone produced by the body or that which was once obtained from the adrenal glands of steers. This potency is also a drawback for long-term treatments. The side effects are, in fact, numerous and detrimental: lowered immune defenses, decalcification of the bones, thinning of the skin, stomach irritation, weight gain, water retention, high blood pressure, diabetes, abnormal distribution of fats throughout the body, and more.

When its pharmaceutical form is used, cortisone will replace the cortisone naturally produced by the body. While its effectiveness is undeniable and it has helped countless patients, its use is a delicate matter. An alternative solution would be to stimulate the body to produce more of its own cortisone. Because it is produced by the body, this cortisone does not cause any unwelcome side effects. A variety of plants (see chapter 5) permit this stimulation. Of course its effect is not as powerful. It does, however, provide enormous assistance without any of the negative side effects listed above.

THE ANTI-INFLAMMATORY OMEGA-3s

The importance of omega-3 fatty acids is a relatively recent discovery. During the second half of the twentieth century, extensive research was performed on essential fatty acids, among others by Russian physician Catherine Kousmine (1904–1992). During this time essential fatty acids were known as F vitamins. That name was eventually dropped as it became known that the quantity of vitamin F needed by the body was on the order of several grams a day, rather than the several milligrams or less that is generally the case with vitamins.

Doctor Catherine Kousmine

A native of Russia, Dr. Kousmine emigrated to Switzerland with her entire family while still a child. She pursued her medical studies in Lausanne, where she split her time between her medical practice and her research. Her studies led her to the discovery of the cause-and-effect relationship between nutritional deficiencies and the onset of disease. Among other things, she demonstrated the importance of essential polyunsaturated fatty acids, which she dubbed F vitamins. As a deficiency of these vitamins was the basic cause of degenerative diseases like cancer, multiple sclerosis, and chronic arthritis, she recommended daily consumption of "Budwig cream," a blend of cottage cheese, flaxseed oil, ground seeds, lemon juice, and nuts. This cream was not a miracle cure; it was simply a means of making sure patients fulfilled their daily requirement for vitamin F as well as other nutrients the body needs.

Kousmine's treatment methods, which have proven to be highly effective, are explained in her books *Soyez bien dans votre assiette* (Eat Right to Feel Right) and *Sauvez votre corps* (Protect Your Body), as well as in various books written by her disciples, for example *La méthode Kousmine* (The Kousmine Method) and *Les 5 piliers de la santé* (The 5 Pillars of Health) (Jouvence Editions).

Among the many properties of the various essential fatty acids—including the omega-3s, the omega-6s, and so on—are the anti-inflammatory effects of the omega-3s. These substances produce the "prostaglandins of peace" described earlier, whose actions counter those of the pro-inflammatory prostaglandins responsible for inflammation.

Anti-inflammatory remedies like plants, aspirin, and cortisone take effect by blocking the activity of pro-inflammatory prostaglandins. Normally the anti-inflammatory prostaglandins would perform this blocking work. Why wouldn't this occur? It is because these prostaglandins are not present or are produced only in quantities too small to be effective. It so happens that their production is entirely dependent on nutritional factors.

Prostaglandins, whether pro- or anti-inflammatory, are constructed by the body from essential fatty acids. The term *essential* underscores the fact that these fatty acids must be supplied by diet, because the body is incapable of synthesizing them itself. When diet supplies an adequate amount of omega-3s, the body easily produces the anti-inflammatory prostaglandins it needs and can control inflammation on its own.

The situation changes totally when omega-3s are not supplied to the body in sufficient quantity. The body is prevented from producing anti-inflammatory prostaglandins because it is missing the elements that are indispensable for that production. It will therefore be unequipped to control inflammations. This state of omega-3 deficiency is quite common today because most people rarely or seldom eat the foods that are good sources of omega-3s.

A deficiency in omega-3s is of even greater concern given that the production of pro-inflammatory prostaglandins depends on other essential fatty acids that, in contrast, are abundant in the

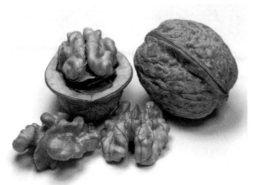

Walnuts are an important source of omega-3 essential fatty acids.

modern diet, and consequently the conditions for their production are quite favorable. The disparity between the different types of essential fatty acids in the diet accentuates the existing imbalance between anti-inflammatory and pro-inflammatory prostaglandins.

GOOD SOURCES OF OMEGA-3s	
First- and Cold-Pressed Oils	**Fatty Fishes**
Camelina	Anchovy
Canola	Halibut
Flax	Herring
Hemp	Mackerel
Soy	Salmon
Walnut	Sardine
Wheat germ	
Other sources: Seaweed or algae like spirulina	

The fatty acids necessary for the production of pro-inflammatory prostaglandins are primarily linoleic acid and arachidonic acid, both omega-6 essential fatty acids. Linoleic acid is abundantly present in commonly consumed oils like corn, sunflower, and peanut. Arachidonic acid is found in products containing animal fats: meats, cheeses, eggs, butter, and so on. A person who regularly eats meat and cheese—which is a vast part of the population—is consequently supplying his or her body with a large number of the substances necessary to produce the prostaglandins that cause inflammation. Because of their substantial presence in the body, it can react quite strongly against any aggression. Its defensive reactions will be quick, strong, and lasting, because it has everything it needs to defend itself. People who are equipped in this way are likely to have easily triggered inflammations that take severe forms—sometimes too severe—and are difficult to stop. The lack of omega-3s and anti-inflammatory prostaglandins prevents the body from putting up any effective resistance to the inflammatory response of the other prostaglandins.

It may seem surprising that nature offers so few foods containing omega-3s. It could even provide grounds for suspecting that nature is not as perfect and well-orchestrated as is commonly alleged. This, however, is not the case. The foods I have mentioned as sources of omega-3s are simply those that have the richest concentrations of this fatty acid. Omega-3s actually can be found in many other foods, just in smaller quantities, though when added together those smaller quantities are adequate to provide for the body's needs. If despite all these food sources an omega-3 deficiency exists, it comes from the fact that these foods (oil-rich seeds, vegetables, and so on) are lacking in the modern diet, and that today's imbalanced, pro-inflammatory diet greatly increases our need for omega-3s. While in 1900 the per capita consumption of meat averaged just 10 pounds or less per year, the current consumption of meat is now around 200 pounds a year per person in the United States, while in France it is 175 pounds. Switzerland is more moderate but still high at 130 pounds per capita.

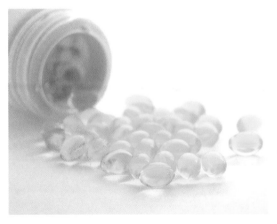

Omega-3 gel caps have found their place in the market of natural supplements.

One aspect of anti-inflammatory therapy therefore consists of giving the body the omega-3s it needs to produce anti-inflammatory prostaglandins. This requires a healthy, balanced diet and omega-3 supplements (see chapter 6).

CONCLUSION

Increasing the body's supply of omega-3s is effective primarily against chronic inflammations, rather than acute ones, because it takes the body some time to increase its production of anti-inflammatory prostaglandins. Once they have been produced, however, they head right into battle against their pro-inflammatory counterparts in order to calm the inflammation. So the anti-inflammatory action of omega-3s is slower than that of medicinal plants or pharmaceuticals like aspirin and cortisone. In these remedies the anti-inflammatory substances are already formed and go directly to work as soon as they enter the body.

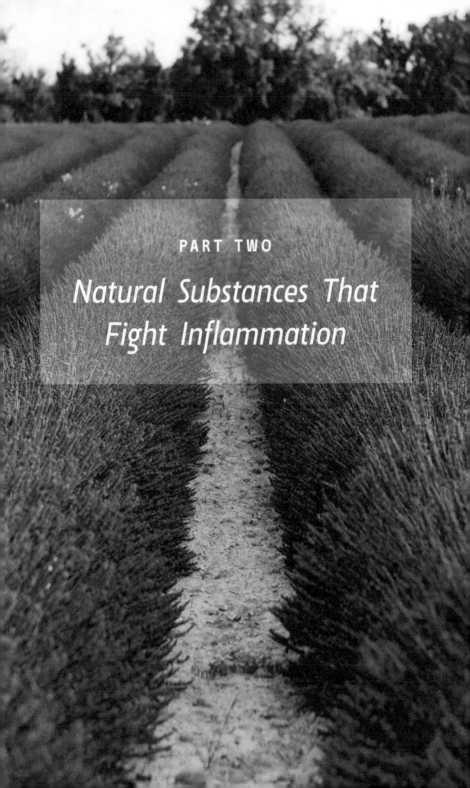

PART TWO

Natural Substances That Fight Inflammation

The natural substances that fight inflammation introduced in this part of the book can be divided into several categories:

1. The first consists of medicinal plants. They come primarily from Europe and America but also from Africa and Asia. They have been selected based on their effectiveness in treating the most common inflammatory diseases.
2. A second category is formed by dietary supplements. One part consists of omega-3s, the essential fatty acids that help the body produce anti-inflammatory prostaglandins. The second part is made up of alkaline supplements. They contain alkaline minerals that generally neutralize the acids that contribute to triggering and maintaining inflammations.
3. The third category consists of various hydrotherapy methods using cold water. Cold water, in fact, has a rapid and powerful anti-inflammatory effect.

The natural anti-inflammatory substances of these three categories have all been used with success to treat inflammation. No one of them is clearly superior to the others; each brings something in its own way, which is different from the others. The important thing in any case is which one or more of them best meets the patient's needs.

It is possible—and often desirable—to use anti-inflammatories from all three categories at the same time.

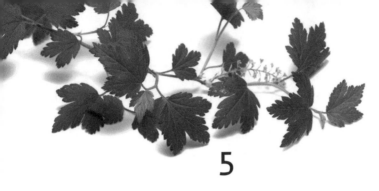

5

Eighteen
Anti-Inflammatory Plants

Cortisone Stimulators, Inflammation Blockers, and Antihistamines

Numerous medicinal plants are effective against inflammation. Those presented here are known for being highly effective and easy to use. They can be divided into three major groups.

1. The first group includes the plants that stimulate the body to produce hormones that reduce or remove inflammation. These anti-inflammatory hormones are members of the cortisone family, for which reason these plants are described as having "cortisone-like" action.
2. The second group consists of plants that work by directly supplying the body with substances that block the inflammatory process.
3. The third group contains plants that have an antihistamine effect. The inflammation mediators—in other words the substances that trigger inflammation—consist not solely

of pro-inflammatory prostaglandins but include a good many others. Among them, histamine figures prominently. It is involved in allergic inflammatory disorders like hay fever, for example. As their name indicates, these antihistaminic plants reduce blood histamine levels, and thereby the inflammation. The other anti-inflammatory plants do not do this; they act on the effects of histamine, but not on its concentration in the body.

The profiles of the plants in these three groups are broken down into subsections that make it possible to easily find the information you are looking for.

The Different Subsections

Name of the Plant: In English and Latin, for correct identification of the plant.

Botanical Description: The appearance and prominent characteristics of the plant.

History: Observations about the plant's use through history.

Part Used: The part of the plant used to make the anti-inflammatory remedies.

Active Principles: The primary constituents that give the plant its anti-inflammatory properties.

Properties: Properties of the plant that are useful to know in making a choice; this list is far from exhaustive.

Target Organs: The organs for which the plant has demonstrated its most effective anti-inflammatory action.

Indications: The illnesses for which the anti-inflammatory properties of the plant are most helpful; this is not an exhaustive list.

Use/Dosage: The form in which the plant should be used.

There can be one or several, depending on the case. These forms are:

Tea: Boiling water is poured over the plant matter (leaves, flowers, and so on). The plant is left to steep for ten minutes, during which time the steaming water will extract the plant's active principles.

Mother tincture: This remedy is obtained by macerating the plant matter in alcohol, in a precise ratio of 10 percent plant matter to 90 percent alcohol.

Glycerin maceration: This remedy is obtained in the same way as the mother tincture, but in a blend of alcohol, glycerin, and water. It is generally used for new-growth plant tissues (buds, rootlets, young sprouts, and so on). It also requires a ratio of 10 percent plant matter to 90 percent liquid.

Capsules: The selected plant is carefully dried and finely ground into a powder. A precise quantity of this powder is then placed inside a capsule.

Essential oil: This is a remedy consisting of the aromatic and volatile oily principles of certain medicinal plants.

Contraindications: Any condition that makes it inadvisable to use the plant being profiled.

You should be able to find the plants described over the following pages at any shop that sells herbs or health products. There you should be able to get more advice on these plants and how to use them and in what doses. The dosage information provided here is generalized and should be tailored for the individual. For example, the dosage may need to be raised or lowered depending on the intensity of the inflammation. And some people may be able to tolerate only one-half to one-fourth of the recommended dosage. Other people may need a higher-than-average dose to get any results. The dosage of capsules can be difficult to calculate, as the quantity of powder they contain will vary from one manufacturer to the next. The recommended dosages provided here are the most common, but you should also refer to the manufacturer's instructions.

Special Notes Concerning Essential Oils

Essential oils are highly concentrated and can sometimes be extremely harsh on the skin and mucous membranes. Diluting them is therefore advisable, and users should start with small doses to test their personal tolerance for each essential oil. For external use a carrier oil is recommended for dilution, and sunflower oil is a good choice. For internal use dilute essential oils in honey or a cold-pressed oil like sunflower or canola. However, because essential oils are so strong, they should only be ingested for a time frame of three to seven days—in other words, during the acute phase of the inflammation.

PLANTS THAT STIMULATE CORTISONE PRODUCTION

+ Black currant
+ Black spruce
+ Scotch pine

The plants of this group have a "cortisone-like" effect; in other words they stimulate the adrenal glands to produce more cortisone. This hormone will then flow at higher levels in the bloodstream and work its anti-inflammatory effect throughout the body. Since this cortisone is produced by the body and is a natural physiological product, it is entirely beneficial, without any adverse side effects.

Black Currant
(Ribes nigrum)

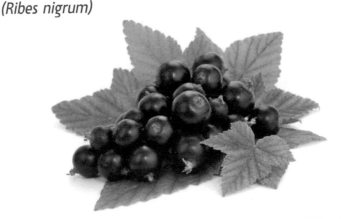

Botanical Description: The black currant is a small bush that can grow to more than 4 feet tall. It produces small, black spherical fruits.

History: Black currant leaves have been used for several centuries for their antiarthritic properties. In the twentieth century, black currant buds were found to contain concentrated levels of these same properties. The recommended preparations are glycerin maceration or mother tincture.

Parts Used: Buds, leaves

Active Principles: Bioflavonoids

Properties:
- Adrenal stimulant
- Powerful anti-inflammatory
- Diuretic

Target Organs: All organs, particularly the respiratory tract and joints

Indications:
Respiratory tract: Hay fever, allergies to dust and animal hair, allergenic asthma

Joints: Acute and chronic arthritis
Urinary tract: Cystitis, prostatitis
General inflammation: Hives, hemorrhoids, et cetera

Use/Dosage:

Glycerin maceration or mother tincture (buds): Take 30 to 50 drops
with water three times a day before mealtime. For hay fever
and other seasonal allergies, maintain this dosage throughout
the season when the pollen to which you are sensitive is present. In the event of an isolated attack, take 50 drops in a glass
of water at once. You should start feeling its effects within
half an hour.

Herbal tea: Pour 1 cup of boiling water over 10 grams of dried
leaves, and let steep for fifteen minutes. Drink 2 or 3 cups a
day. The tea's effect is primarily antiarthritic and diuretic; it
is not antiallergic.

Black Spruce
(Picea mariana)

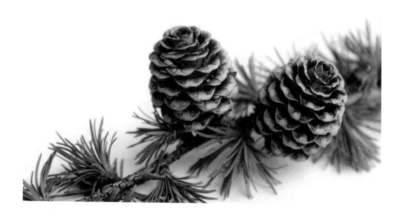

Botanical Description: Black spruce is a fir tree, one of almost
forty members of the genus *Picea* found primarily in the world's
northern temperate and boreal regions. It is one of the most

cold-tolerant trees of this genus. It grows mainly in Canada, up to the very borders of the tundra.

History: Black spruce provides a very solid wood for carpentry. Its buds and needles are rich in vitamin C. They were once used to brew spruce beer, which was used to prevent scurvy.

Part Used: Needles from the young branches

Active Principles: Terpenes, bornyl acetate

Properties:
- Adrenal stimulant
- Anti-inflammatory
- Antimicrobial
- Overall stimulant

Target Organs: Adrenal glands and the respiratory tract

Indications:
Respiratory tract: Rhinitis (the common cold), rhinopharyngitis, sinusitis, bronchitis, coughs, hay fever, asthma
Urinary tract: Prostatitis
Digestive tract: Candida enteritis, parasites

Use/Dosage: Black spruce is primarily used in the form of essential oil.
Orally: Take 1 drop of essential oil in honey or cold-pressed oil three times a day.
Skin application: Use 1 to 3 drops of essential oil per ½ teaspoon of sunflower or another carrier oil. Massage onto the back, around the area of the adrenal glands (around the upper kidneys at the level of the bottom ribs).

Scotch Pine
(Pinus sylvestris)

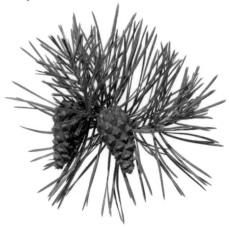

Botanical Description: The Scotch pine is a coniferous tree that grows in the cold and mountainous regions of Europe and Asia. It can grow to 100 feet in height. It is very resistant to frost but requires a lot of sunlight. Its bark is dark and scaly, except toward the top of the tree, where it is flaky and orange. Its needles, which are grouped in pairs, are deep green in color. It gives off a pleasant pine odor. The species name *sylvestris* is based on the Latin *sylva,* meaning "forest."

History: The young needles are harvested for their therapeutic properties. They are often sold under the (incorrect) name of spruce buds.

Parts Used: Needles, buds

Active Principles: Various terpenes

Properties:
- Adrenal stimulant
- Anti-inflammatory
- Anti-infectious
- Overall stimulant

Target Organs: The entire body

Indications:
Respiratory tract: Sinusitis, bronchitis
Joints: Arthritis in general
Urinary tract: Cystitis, prostatitis

Use/Dosage:
Herbal tea: Pour 1 quart of boiling water over 20 to 50 grams of buds and let steep for ten minutes. Drink 3 cups a day.
Mother tincture: Take 10 to 20 drops diluted in a little water three times a day.
Essential oil: Take 3 drops in honey or cold-pressed oil three or four times a day.
Capsules: Take 2 capsules three times a day when inflammation comes on, and then 2 capsules two times a day until it has completely cleared.

Contraindications: Avoid Scotch pine in cases of high blood pressure, nervousness, or weak kidneys.

PLANTS THAT BLOCK INFLAMMATION MEDIATORS

+ Basil
+ Bay laurel
+ Devil's claw
+ Eyebright
+ Lavender
+ Lemon eucalyptus
+ Meadowsweet
+ Roman chamomile
+ Turmeric
+ White willow
+ Wintergreen
+ Propolis

These plants possess substances that block or curb the activity of the mediators (triggers) of inflammation.

Basil
(Ocimum basilicum)

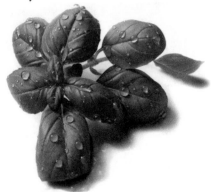

Botanical Description: Basil grows in clumps of stems that range from 8 to 20 inches in height. The leaves are an intense light green and the flowers small and white. This plant gives off a strong and pleasant odor. While native to the tropics, it now grows throughout the world.

History: The word *basil* comes from the Greek *basilikon,* meaning "royal." The plant is regarded as a royal remedy. It relieves tension and offers great assistance in all disorders affecting the digestive tract. Basil is also a popular culinary herb used in everything from salads and soups to meat dishes and pastas (especially the famous Italian pesto).

Parts Used: Flowering tops, leaves

Active Principle: Chavicol

Properties:
- Extremely potent anti-inflammatory
- Powerful antispasmodic
- Powerful antiviral

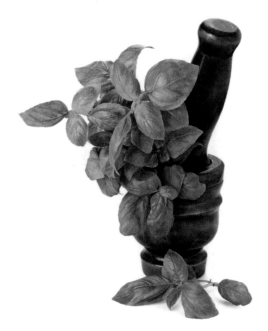

Target Organs: Digestive tract, nerves, urinary tract, joints

Indications:

Digestive tract: Gastritis, heartburn and acidic stomach, enteritis, colitis, diarrhea, spasms, et cetera

Nerves: Neuritis

Urinary tract: Cystitis, prostatitis

Joints: Arthritis, tendinitis

Use/Dosage:

Herbal tea: Pour 1 cup boiling water over 3 to 4 fresh leaves and let steep for ten minutes. Drink 3 or 4 cups a day.

Essential oil: Take 1 or 2 drops in honey or cold-pressed oil three times a day, for a maximum of five days.

☝ Good to Know

Basil leaves lose their healing properties when dried.

Bay Laurel
(Laurus nobilis)

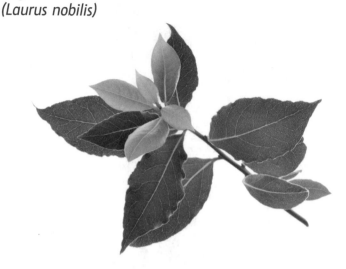

Botanical Description: Bay laurel, also called Grecian laurel or true laurel, is a small tree with beautiful evergreen leaves whose upper surface is shiny. In spring it produces small white flowers, which then produce small black berries the size of a cherry.

History: In ancient Greece the laurel was said to be sacred to the god Apollo and symbolized glory. Crowns woven of its branches were placed on the heads of heroes. Bay leaves are used as a culinary seasoning, not only giving dishes good flavor but also stimulating digestion. The oil of bay laurel fruits is thick and almost solid; it is the source of "laurel butter," which is used as a rub to treat arthritis.

⚠ Caution!

Do not confuse bay laurel with the garden plants rose laurel (oleander) or cherry laurel; they are poisonous.

Part Used: Leaves

Active Principle: Costunolide

Properties:

- Anti-inflammatory
- Powerful analgesic
- Antispasmodic
- Anti-infectious
- Nervine/nerve harmonizer

Target Organs: Respiratory tract (nose, sinuses, throat, lungs), digestive tract (liver, small intestine, colon), mouth, skin, joints, muscles, nerves

Indications:

Respiratory tract: Sinusitis, rhinitis, pharyngitis, rhinopharyngitis, laryngitis, bronchitis, asthma

Digestive tract: Diarrhea, enteritis, colitis, gastroenteritis

Mouth: Tonsillitis, gingivitis, glossitis, canker sores, dental pain, periodontitis, abscess

Skin: Acne, eczema, boils, cracks, ulcer, hives, whitlow

Joints and muscles: Arthritis, osteoarthritis, gout, lumbago

Nerves: Sciatica, neuritis

Use/Dosage: The simplest means of using this plant is to use its essential oil.

Orally: Take 1 or 2 drops of laurel essential oil in honey or cold-pressed oil two or three times a day.

Skin application (undiluted): You can use bay laurel essential oil neat, or undiluted, on a skin eruption or inflammation. Apply 1 drop on a pimple, abscess, or canker sore three or four times a day. For a larger area, apply 2 or 3 drops three or four times a day.

Skin application (diluted): Mix 10 drops of essential oil in 1 teaspoon of sunflower or another carrier oil. Massage this into the affected area three or four times a day.

Gargle: Mix 2 or 3 drops of essential oil in a little milk, and stir that into a half-full glass of water. Gargle three or four times a day.

Bath: Mix 15 to 20 drops of the essential oil in 1 tablespoon of milk and add to a bathtub full of water.

➕ Expert Tips and Tricks

Some people are not able to tolerate the essential oil of laurel very well. Consequently, a little skin test is essential before using it. Put a drop of essential oil on the skin at the fold of the elbow. If no irritation or redness appears after two or three hours, there is no intolerance. In the opposite case, it is better not to use this oil.

Devil's Claw
(Harpagophytum procumbens)

Botanical Description: This is a low-lying plant whose fruits are equipped with long, curved hooklike growths. Hence the plant's name: *harpago* in Latin means "hook," and *phytum* means "plant." In other words "the plant with hooks." As is the case with many plants, the purpose of these hooks is to aid in the dissemination and propagation of the plant. When they become stuck in the feet and fur of animals, the seeds are carried far. However, the hardened nature of these hooks injures the soft portions of the hooves of livestock, which can lead to infection and disease, and so the plant's origin was attributed to the devil.

History: Devil's claw is native to the hot, dry regions of southern Africa. It grows in South Africa and in the Kalahari Desert that bestrides Namibia and Botswana. The inhabitants of this region use it to treat many health problems, particularly arthritic pain.

Westerners discovered the medicinal virtues of devil's claw

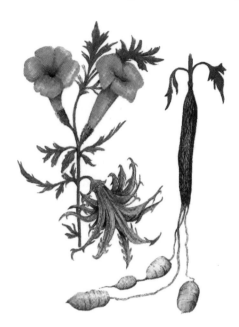

in the early 1900s, and it has been used since that time in Europe and America. Studies conducted to pinpoint its properties offer evidence of this plant's great effectiveness against inflammatory disorders, which has caused its popularity to boom. Today it is among the bestselling medicinal plants in the world.

Part Used: Root

Active Principle: Harpagoside

Properties:
- Powerful anti-inflammatory; several studies have shown it to be as effective as the various anti-inflammatory pharmaceuticals

Target Organs: Joints, muscles, tendons

Indications:
Joints: Arthritis, osteoarthitis, gout
Muscles: Back pain, lumbago
Nerves: Sciatica, neuritis
Tendons: Tendinitis

Use/Dosage:

Herbal tea: It is possible to make an infusion of devil's claw, but its bitterness is an obstacle to the regular and sufficient consumption of the tea.

Mother tincture: Take 20 to 30 drops in a little water three times a day.

Capsules: Capsules or tablets of the powdered root are the most common and practical means of use. Follow the manufacturer's instructions, which generally instruct users to take 1 or 2 capsules or tablets three times a day, with food.

Contraindications: Avoid devil's claw in cases of gastric or duodenal ulcer.

✛ Expert Tips and Tricks

The anti-inflammatory effect of devil's claw will manifest quickly (in one to two days) and will be evident by the reduction of pain. But a profound effect will only be obtained after several weeks, or even months, of regular use of the plant. It is generally recommended to take devil's claw for two or three months and to repeat as needed.

Eyebright
(Euphrasia officinalis)

Botanical Description: Eyebright is a small, low-lying plant that grows in pastures at high altitudes. Its small, pretty flowers are white with a yellow spot and striped with violet. It is semi-parasitic, relying on the root structure of nearby plants for part of its sustenance.

History: Theophrastus (fourth century BCE) and Dioscorides (first century CE) recommended eyebright for the treatment of eye problems. Hildegard von Bingen gave similar counsel in the

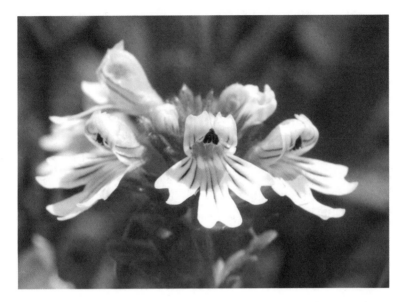

Middle Ages. Today it is still one of the standard plants—along with bachelor's button (*Centaurea cyanus*)—used for treating eye inflammations. Its beneficial effects have earned it nicknames like "glasses breaker" and "myopia herb." In Germany it is called *augentrost,* or "consolation for the eyes." These virtues can also be seen in its English name.

Part Used: The entire flowering part of the plant

Active Principle: Aucubin

Properties:
- Anti-inflammatory
- Analgesic

Target Organs: Eyes, nasal mucous membranes

Indications:
Eyes: Conjunctivitis, blepharitis, keratitis, sty
Nose: Infectious colds and hay fever with heavy mucous discharge

Use/Dosage: Eyebright is used primarily externally in the form of compresses, washes, and eyebaths.

Compress: Boil a handful of dried plant matter in 1 quart of water for ten minutes; then remove from the heat and let it steep for ten more minutes. Let cool. Soak cotton pads in the infused liquid, place them over your eyes, and relax for ten minutes. Repeat several times a day.

Nasal wash: To anesthetize and reduce inflammation in the nasal mucous membranes during an infectious cold or allergic disorder like hay fever, prepare a decoction as described for the compress above. Fill a bowl with this liquid. Leaning over it, submerge your nose in the liquid. Breathe the liquid into your nose, and then let it drip out into the sink or a separate container. Repeat several times.

⊕ Expert Tips and Tricks

There are many commercially available products made with eyebright and bachelor's button. They can be used to bathe the eyes. These products often include a small cup for facilitating the bath.

Lavender
(Lavandula angustifolia)

Botanical Description: Lavender is a very well-known plant. It rises in numerous thin stems at whose tips bloom spikes of extremely aromatic blue-violet flowers.

History: The word *lavender* comes from the Latin *lavare,* meaning "to wash" or "to clean." Was this plant so named because Romans added it to their bathwater or because washerwomen added it their laundry as perfume? Or could it even have been because of its calming, antispasmodic properties, which help us relax and "wash away" our cares? Lavender is praised by all for its many virtues; Jean Valnet described it as "the most valuable"

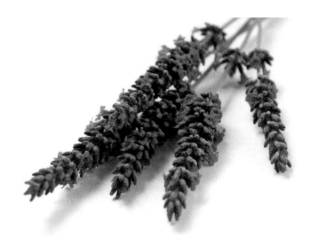

of plants, and French author B. Saint-Girons called it "the first and foremost of the essential oils." It has been heralded as being good for just about everything.

Part Used: Flowering tops

Active Principles: Linalyl acetate, linalool, and more than three hundred other substances, which makes lavender one of the most richly provided medicinal plants—hence its many virtues

Properties:
- Generally anti-inflammatory
- Calming
- Analgesic
- Antispasmodic

Target Organs: Skin, respiratory tract, digestive tract

Indications:

Skin: Acne, burns, sunburn, cracking, abrasions, eczema, eruptive fever, bites, insect stings, infected wounds, pruritis, redness, hives, whitlow

Respiratory tract: Bronchitis, asthma, nagging cough, sore throat

Digestive tract: Diarrhea, enteritis

Various: Muscle aches, joint pains, toothache, otitis, cystitis

Use/Dosage: Lavender is primarily used as an essential oil. This oil is quite gentle and can be applied directly to the skin.

Orally: Take 3 to 5 drops diluted in honey or cold-pressed oil three times a day.

Skin application: Apply 1 to 15 drops, depending on the size of the surface to be treated, three times a day. Spread the drops over the affected area and lightly massage them to help the oil enter the tissues.

Bath: Mix 15 to 20 drops of the essential oil in 1 tablespoon of milk or some other bath-worthy liquid, and add to a bathtub full of water.

 Good to Know

By itself lavender's anti-inflammatory property is not the most powerful one among medicinal plants, but it is reinforced by many other of lavender's properties. Lavender also has, for example, an analgesic, calming action that increases fluid flow, facilitates wound healing, lowers blood pressure, and counters infection and spasm. This makes it one of the most valuable agents for dealing with inflammation.

Lemon Eucalyptus
(Corymbia citriodora)

Botanical Description: Lemon eucalyptus is one of the six hundred species in the large eucalyptus family. They are large trees with smooth trunks that grow rapidly. Their thin, long leaves are rich with active principles. The lemon eucalyptus takes its name from its strong lemony aroma.

History: A native of Australia, lemon eucalyptus was widely introduced into the Americas and Europe in the latter half of the nineteenth century to fill clear cuts, especially in marshy

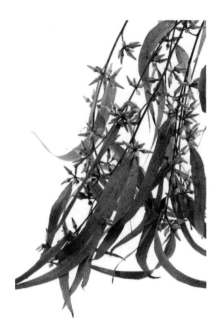

areas. It requires a lot of water, which with its long roots it can remove from large areas of the ground in which it grows. And its strong aromatic odor repels mosquitos, which are endemic in these kinds of environments.

Part Used: Leaves; those found on older branches of the tree have a higher concentration of active principles

Active Principle: Citronella

Properties:
- Anti-inflammatory
- Analgesic

Target Organs: Joints, tendons, muscles, nerves

Indications:
Joints: Arthritis, osteoarthritis, gout
Nerves: Sciatica, shingles
Tendons: Tendinitis, epicondylitis
Muscles: Strains, tears

Blood vessels: Phlebitis, arteritis, hemorrhoids

Skin: Eczema, itching, ringworm, insect stings, whitlow

Use/Dosage: Lemon eucalyptus is used primarily in the form of an essential oil. This oil gives off a strong odor of lemon and eucalyptus.

Orally: Take 3 to 5 drops with honey or cold-pressed oil three to five times a day.

Skin application: Mix 10 drops of the essential oil with 1 teaspoon of sunflower or another carrier oil. Rub this into the affected area three or four times a day, for a maximum of three weeks.

Bath: Mix 15 to 20 drops in 1 tablespoon of milk or some other bath-worthy liquid, and add to a bathtub full of water.

Meadowsweet
(Filipendula ulmaria)

Botanical Description: A plant of meadows with plenty of water, meadowsweet features stems that grow to 50 inches in height and more. In July and August, they are crowned with small, creamy white flowers that are extremely aromatic. This is a beautiful, slender plant that dominates and overshadows everything around it, like a queen—hence another of its common names, queen of the meadow.

History: Meadowsweet has been used since antiquity for its antiarthritic properties. Studies performed on this plant in the nineteenth century led to the discovery of its active principle and the development of aspirin (see page 82).

Part Used: Flowering tops, harvested shortly before the flowers bloom

Active Principle: Salicylic acid

Properties:
- Anti-inflammatory
- Diuretic

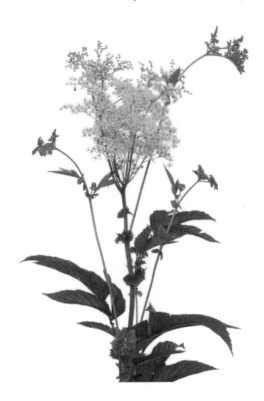

Target Organs: Joints, nerves

Indications:

Joints: Pain, ankylosis, swelling, arthritis, osteoarthritis, gout

Nerves: Neuralgia, neuritis

Tendons: Tendinitis

Use/Dosage:

Herbal tea: Pour 1 cup of boiling water over 1 teaspoon of dried leaves and flowers, and let steep for ten minutes. Drink 3 cups a day. (Note: Do not boil this plant; that will cause it to lose its active principles.)

Capsules: Take 2 capsules three times a day, before meals.

Contraindications: Avoid meadowsweet if you are allergic to aspirin or are taking blood thinners.

Roman Chamomile
(Chamaemelum nobile)

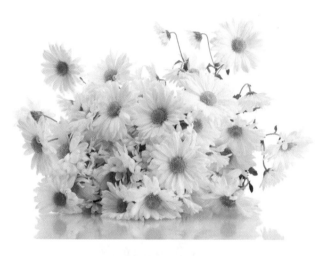

Botanical Description: A small plant that grows from 4 to 12 inches high, chamomile has branches that crawl over the ground before lifting toward the sky. At their tips these heavily branching stems have flowers with white petals around a yellow center. The plant gives off a pleasant and pervasive aroma. Its flavor is slightly bitter and aromatic.

History: The authors of antiquity never mention this variety of chamomile. The oldest known accounts of its use go back only to the sixteenth century. Despite its "youth," it is commonly used against stomach disorders.

Parts Used: Flowers, leafy stems

Active Principles: Isobutyl angelate, pinocarvone

Properties:
- Anti-inflammatory
- Antispasmodic

- Calming
- Analgesic
- Healing (wounds)

Target Organs: Digestive tract, skin, nerves

Indications:

Digestive tract: Gastritis, stomach ulcers, enteritis, colitis

Skin: Eczema, boils, burns, cuts, itching, redness, cracking, hives, whitlow

Nerves: Facial and other neuralgias, painful teething in babies, neuritis

Eyes: Conjunctivitis, blepharitis

Use/Dosage:

Internally:

Herbal tea: Pour 1 cup boiling water over 5 to 10 of the flower heads, and let steep for ten minutes. Drink 3 to 5 cups a day.

Mother tincture: Take 30 drops diluted in a little water three times a day.

Essential oil: Take 2 to 4 drops in honey or cold-pressed oil three or four times a day.

Capsules: Take 2 capsules three times a day with water.

Externally:

For inflammations of the skin and eyes: Pour boiling water over chamomile (1 tablespoon of herb per cup of water), and let steep 10 minutes. (The amount you prepare will be based on the size of the surface to be treated.) Let the infusion cool until it is lukewarm, and then apply as a wash, compress, or bath.

For inflamed nerves: Dilute 3 or 4 drops of chamomile essential oil in ½ teaspoon of sunflower oil, and rub over the afflicted area. Repeat three or four times a day.

Turmeric
(Curcuma longa, C. aromatica)

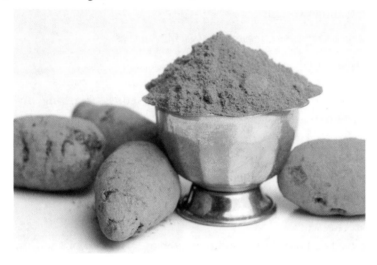

Botanical Description: Turmeric grows in India and throughout Southeast Asia. It is an herbaceous plant with extremely long leaves and a very thick root, which averages about 4 inches in diameter. The root is the part of the plant that is used for medicinal purposes. It is cut into rounds that are put out to dry; it then assumes its orange color and gives off a pleasant aroma. These dried slices are crushed into powder for medicinal and culinary use.

History: Turmeric has been used in Asia for an extremely long time. It is one of the most commonly prescribed plants in traditional Indian and Chinese medicine. When dried and powdered, it provides a highly valued cooking spice; it is one of the ingredients in curry. It imbues foods with a distinctive yellow color. Empirically, the people who used it noticed that turmeric helped foods retain their freshness, flavor, and nutritional value. Modern research has shown that these effects are due to the heavy presence of antioxidants.

Part Used: Root

Active Principle: Curcumin

Properties:

• Anti-inflammatory; studies have shown it to be as effective against arthritis as all the commonly prescribed anti-inflammatory pharmaceuticals

Target Organs: Digestive tract, joints, skin

Indications:

Digestive tract: Gastritis, irritable bowel syndrome, enteritis, colitis

Joints: Arthritis, osteoarthritis

Skin: Wounds, eczema, redness, whitlow

Use/Dosage:

Herbal tea: Pour 1 cup of boiling water over 1 to 5 grams of powdered turmeric, and let steep for ten minutes. Drink 1 to 3 cups a day.

Mother tincture: Take 5 to 20 drops diluted in water two or three times a day.

Capsules: Take 1 or 2 capsules three times a day.

Compress or poultice: Apply a compress (using an infusion) or a poultice (using the powder) of turmeric to the affected area three or four times a day.

White Willow
(Salix alba)

Botanical Description: White willow is one of the two hundred different species of willow trees. The name *willow* comes from the Celtic language and means "near water." This tree grows in fact along waterways and in moist terrain. The *white* in its name comes from the silvery white underside of the tree's leaves. This tree has enormous vitality; just stick a branch in the ground and it will take root and start growing.

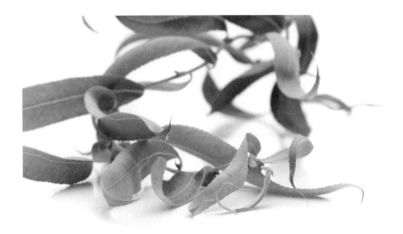

History: The white willow, like other species of willow, has been used since earliest antiquity for its anti-inflammatory properties in the treatment of arthritis and neuralgia. This is one of the plants that contributed to the discovery of aspirin (see page 81).

Part Used: Primarily the bark

Active Principle: Salicin

Properties:

- Anti-inflammatory
- Antispasmodic
- Lowers fever
- Analgesic
- Sedative

Target Organs: Joints, nerves, muscles

Indications:
Joints: Arthritis, gout, back pain
Nerves: Neuralgia, facial neuralgia, sciatica
Muscles: Lumbago

Use/Dosage:
Decoction: Boil 25 to 30 grams of bark in 1 quart of water for

five minutes, then remove from the heat and let steep for ten minutes more. Drink 2 to 3 cups a day.

Capsules: Take 2 capsules three times a day, before eating.

? Did You Know?

Because of its strong potential for calming painful inflammation, Dr. Valnet nicknamed white willow "the pain-fighting tree."

The active substances of willow are the source of aspirin. The latter can irritate the stomach so strongly that it can cause ulcers. You might fear that willow would have the same effect, but that is not at all true. To the contrary willow relieves hyperacidity of the stomach.

Wintergreen
(Gaultheria fragrantissima, G. procumbens)

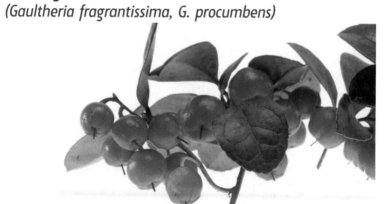

Botanical Description: This is a small, shrubby plant reaching about 5 to 6 inches in height that is in the heather family. *G. procumbens* is native to North America, while *G. fragrantissima* is native to China. Both produce small, edible fruits shaped like apples.

History: Wintergreen was long used by Native Americans to treat inflammation, pains, and fever. They made decoctions from its leaves or simply chewed them directly.

Part Used: Leaves

Active Principle: Methyl salicylate (which comprises 95 to 98 percent of the essential oil)

Properties:

- Anti-inflammatory
- Antispasmodic
- Analgesic

Target Organs: Joints, muscles, tendons, nerves

Indications:
Joints: Acute and chronic arthritis
Muscles: Pain, spasm, strain, lumbago
Tendons: Tendinitis
Nerves: Neuritis, sciatica

Use/Dosage: Wintergreen is primarily used as an essential oil that is diluted and applied to the skin. Use 1 or 2 drops of essential oil per ½ teaspoon of sunflower or another carrier oil. Rub over the afflicted joint or muscles two or three times a day.

Contraindications: Because of its high concentration of active principles, wintergreen is not recommended for individuals taking blood thinners; the accumulation of anticoagulant factors could be too high. It is also contraindicated for people with allergies to salicylic derivatives, like aspirin. It should be avoided by pregnant women and children under the age of six.

 Good to Know

Wintergreen is used in the manufacture of many massage oils and balms for athletes.

Propolis

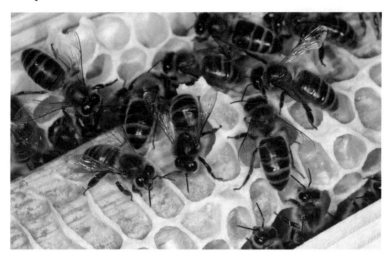

Botanical Description: Propolis is the only anti-inflammatory substance in this chapter that is not a plant. It is, in fact, of both plant and animal origin. Bees prepare it from resinous and gummy substances that they harvest from buds and bark, to which they introduce their own secretions. Bees use propolis to repair cracks and seal off openings in the hive. In addition to its role as an all-purpose putty, it offers protection to the entire hive as a disinfectant.

History: Propolis was used by the ancient Greeks, who gave it its current name: *pro* means "in front," and *polis* means "town" or "city." Propolis in in fact found in large quantity at the entry to the hive, where it is used to build a defensive wall against enemies. In addition to the ancient Greeks, it was also used by the physicians of ancient Rome, the Persian physician Avicenna, and the Incans.

Part Used: Propolis as a whole

Active Principles: Flavonoids, coumarins, various acids, phenols, et cetera

Properties:

- Ant-inflammatory
- Anesthetic (extremely powerful)
- Antimicrobial
- Heals wounds
- Antioxidant

Target Organs: Respiratory tract, mouth, digestive tract, urinary tract, skin

Indications:

Respiratory tract: Rhinitis, sinusitis, otitis, sore throat, laryngitis, tracheitis, bronchitis, asthma, hay fever

Mouth: Gingivitis, glossitis, canker sores, dental pain, periodontitis

Digestive tract: Stomatitis, gastritis, enteritis, colitis

Urinary tract: Cystitis, prostatitis, urethritis

Skin: Abscess, boil, burn, wound, eczema, hives, whitlow, shingles

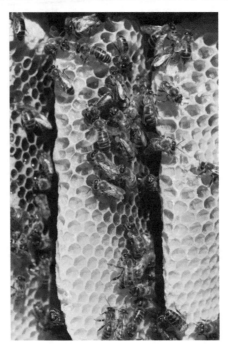

Use/Dosage:

Chewable paste: Take 1 gram three times a day, between meals. Chew it slowly until it dissolves completely. When you start chewing, a burning sensation may appear in your mouth. You'll need to continue this dosage for about a week for it to be effective.

Granulated or powdered: Take 1 gram three times a day, before meals. Take it with a little water, and mix it well with your saliva before swallowing. Take only one dose (1 gram) on the first day, two doses on the second day, and three doses on the third in order to test your tolerance. If you experience no ill effects, continue with the three-time-daily regimen. You'll need to continue this dosage for about a week for it to be effective.

Mother tincture: Take 25 to 50 drops, diluted in water, three times a day.

Skin application: Apply as an ointment to the affected area three or four times a day.

ANTIHISTAMINIC PLANTS

+ Birch
+ Black cumin (also known as nutmeg flower or nigella)
+ English (or pedunculate) oak

Histamines are inflammation mediators, especially when allergies are involved. The plants described here reduce histamine levels in the bloodstream and thereby exert an anti-inflammatory effect.

Histamine is a type of protein. It can be found in small quantities in every cell of the body, but it is present in higher levels in the cells of the tissues most prone to attack and trauma, like those of the skin and mucous membranes.

In the event that a cell is attacked or injured, the histamine it contains spills into the extracellular fluid. When it comes into contact with the surrounding cells, the histamine triggers a defensive reaction similar to the one caused by pro-inflammatory prostaglandins. The capillaries dilate, organs secrete fluids (the tears caused by hay fever), and the smooth muscles spasm (hence the colics). These are all defensive means used by the body to fight the attack.

When histamine is released by many cells at the same time, its presence in the tissues causes damage like a poison. Depending on the individual case, the result can be a dramatic drop in blood pressure (*collapsus*), asthma, hives, colic, or diarrhea.

Birch
(Betula pubescens)

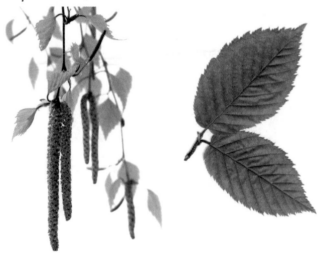

Botanical Description: The birch tree is easily recognized thanks to its distinctive papery white bark, thanks to which it is commonly known as white birch. But this name in fact is bestowed upon a number of birch varieties, of which *Betula pubescens* is but one example. Etymologically speaking, *betula* means "tree" and *pubescens* means "hair." The hairs can be found on the young branches of this species of birch and are not found on the other varieties. This birch is a very undemanding tree with good cold tolerance. It happily colonizes bare and abandoned areas.

History: This tree has been valued throughout history for its medicinal virtues.

Parts Used: Leaves, sap, buds

Active Principles: Hyperoside, betuloside

Properties:
- Antihistaminic (buds)
- Diuretic
- Lowers fever
- Antiarthritic

Target Organs: Overall body tissues, respiratory tract, joints

Indications:
Respiratory tract: Hay fever, allergies to dust and animal hair, allergic asthma
Joints: Arthritis, gout

Use/Dosage:
Glycerin maceration: Take 30 drops of the gemmotherapy remedy *Betula pubescens* buds 1D (a glycerin and alcohol extract diluted in a 1:10 ratio with water) with water three times a day.

Black Cumin
(Nigella sativa)

Botanical Description: This widely cultivated nigella is an annual of some 14 to 20 inches in height that is distinguished by its feathery leaves, in other words leaves that are cut into narrow threads or lashes, creating an intricate tangle. Its flowers are blue and its seeds are deep gray to black, from which its name of black cumin arises (though it has nothing in common with the cumin used in Indian and North African cuisine). It is now also widely referred to as nigella or nutmeg flower.

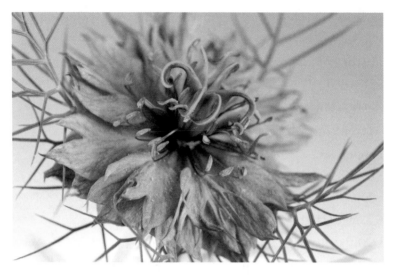

History: This plant is cultivated in the East and in central Europe for its seeds. These seeds have a bitter, burning taste and are widely used to impart flavor to breads and the string cheeses that can be found in eastern European and Jewish delicatessens. In Germany they are used to make pancakes, among other dishes, to which they impart a peppery taste. The seeds' antihistaminic properties were discovered only recently, but they have quickly become one of the primary herbal remedies for lowering blood histamine levels.

Part Used: Seeds

Active Principle: Nigellone

Properties:
• Antihistaminic

Target Organs: Respiratory tract, blood vessels of the head

Indications:
Respiratory tract: Hay fever, allergies, allergic asthma
Blood vessels: Headaches, migraines

Use/Dosage:
Mother tincture: Take 10 to 30 drops in water, three times a day.

English Oak
(Quercus robur; syn. *Q. pedunculata)*

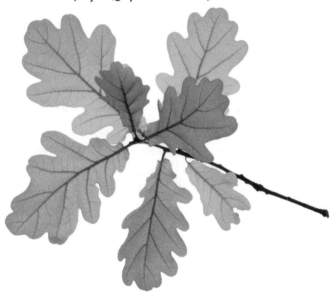

Botanical Description: This familiar tree can be recognized by its sessile leaves that are carved into several pairs of rounded lobes. It can reach heights ranging from 120 to 160 feet and can live to be seven hundred to eight hundred years old.

This species of oak is sometimes called pedunculate oak in reference to the fact that, in contrast to other species, it bears its acorns and flowers at the end of long stalks or peduncles. Its wood is extremely hard and resistant to rot.

History: English oak's massive branches give it an air of strength and solidity, and perhaps for this reason, it has been revered throughout history. In ancient Greece it was said to be the tree sacred to Zeus. In the time of the Celts, Druids performed their ceremonies at the foot of an oak tree.

Parts Used: Buds, leaves, young bark

Active Principles: Quercetin, quercitol

Properties:

- Antihistaminic (buds)
- Astringent (bark, leaves)
- Tonic

Target Organ: The body's tissues, respiratory tract

Indications:

Respiratory tract: Hay fever, allergies, allergic asthma

Use/Dosage:

Glycerin maceration: Take 35 drops of the gemmotherapy remedy *Quercus pedunculata* buds 1D (a glycerin and alcohol extract diluted in a 1:10 ratio with water) with water three times a day, before meals.

⊕ Expert Tips and Tricks

A basic treatment for an allergic terrain consists of combining the effects of birch and oak. You should take 50 drops of birch glycerin macerate (*Betula pubescens* buds 1D) at noon and 50 drops of oak glycerin macerate (*Quercus pedunculata* buds 1D) in the evening.

CONCLUSION

Nature offers such a vast array of plants with anti-inflammatory properties that I could introduce only a small selection here. Depending on the patient's constitution, some will have greater effects than others. It is up to each patient to try out these plants in order to find which is most appropriate for him or her.

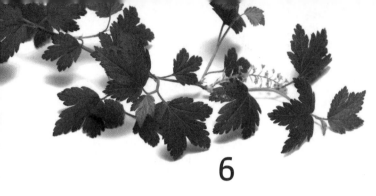

6

Supplements and Diets for Fighting Inflammation

Omega-3s and Alkaline Minerals

Two kinds of dietary supplements help calm inflammations by virtue of the nutrients they contain. The first kind are supplements of omega-3 fatty acids of plant or animal (fish) origin; the second comprise a base of alkaline minerals. These latter, by neutralizing excess acids in the tissues, reduce inflammations and can even prevent them from being triggered.

THE OMEGA-3s

Omega-3 fatty acids have an anti-inflammatory effect because they permit the body to produce the prostaglandins that naturally soothe inflammation. Our ability to produce these anti-inflammatory prostaglandins is directly dependent on the omega-3 content of the foods we consume. Unfortunately, the modern diet is dramatically lacking in these essential substances.

Our daily intake of omega-3s should equal about 2 grams. In practice, though, in today's typical diet the omega-3 intake falls in the range of 0.2 to 0.6 gram a day, which gives us only 10 to 30 percent of what the body actually requires. Thus, when inflammation occurs, the body does not have enough omega-3s on hand to fight it.

⚠ Caution!

Omega-3s have a blood-thinning effect that can combine with and exaggerate the effects of pharmaceutical blood thinners. If you are taking blood thinners, consult your doctor to determine a safe level of omega-3 intake.

In order to give it the tools it needs to effectively defend itself against inflammation, the body should therefore be generously supplied with omega-3s, which will begin to accumulate in its tissues. This physiological process cannot be achieved overnight, however, but is one that extends over time. This explains why supplementing with omega-3s does not show immediate results. Several weeks, or even months, depending on the scale of the existing deficiency, can elapse before any effect appears.

Once the deficiency has been addressed, it is still necessary to meet the body's daily need for 2 grams or more of omega-3s.

Diet is key to our supply of omega-3s. The body cannot manufacture them itself, or if it does, it is with great difficulty and in quantities that are too small to perform any meaningful function. Numerous foods contain omega-3s, some in small quantities and others in much larger proportions. These latter are the ones that interest us here.

The Anti-Inflammation Diet

While taking omega-3 supplements can be helpful, it is also necessary to follow a diet that provides a generous omega-3 intake. The basic principles of such an anti-inflammation diet can be seen in the following examples:

Proteins

Consume liberally:

- Fatty fish: mackerel, herring, salmon, sardines, anchovies, trout, eel, etc.
- Eggs
- Legumes: lentils, broad beans, white beans, etc.

Consume in moderation:

- Meats
- Cheeses

Carbohydrates

Consume liberally:

- Whole-grain or brown rice
- Whole-grain pastas
- Potatoes

Consume in moderation:

- Other grains
- Bread
- Cereal flakes

Fats

Consume liberally:

- Canola or flaxseed oil
- Almonds, walnuts, flaxseeds

Vegetables

- Eat as much of any vegetable you please, especially leafy green vegetables (lettuce, arugula, cabbage, kale)

Fruits

- Eat all the fruits and as much as you please

Spices

- Use spices diversely and liberally: garlic, onion, parsley, chives, etc.

👆 **Good to Know**

Many different fatty acids are classified as omega-3s. The primary ones are:

- Alpha-linolenic acid (ALA)
- Eicosapentaenoic acid (EPA)
- Docosahexaenoic acid (DHA)

Because omega-3s are fatty acids, they belong to the large family of lipids. So it should come as no surprise that their most generous sources can be found in lipid-rich foods of plant or animal origin.

Plant Sources of Omega-3s

The highest concentrations of lipids in plants can be found in their seeds. Oil can be obtained by pressing these seeds. Obviously, only cold-pressed oils will be good sources of omega-3s, as heat destroys these fatty acids.

The table on the facing page lists commonly available vegetable oils that are rich sources of omega-3s. The distinguishing features and dosages for each of these oils will be discussed in the text following the table.

Canola, soy, and walnut oils must be ingested in relatively large amounts, from 1 to several tablespoons, in order to supply the body with sufficient omega-3s. Canola and soy oils are fairly common and inexpensive. They can easily be used to make salad dressings or added to vegetables and other dishes (after cooking, to preserve their omega-3 content).

The other oils—wheat germ, flax, hemp, camelina, and perilla—are not in such common use. They command a higher price but can be taken in smaller quantities, anywhere from 1 teaspoon to 1 tablespoon.

VEGETABLE OILS RICHEST IN OMEGA-3s	
Oil	Omega-3 Content
Perilla (shiso)	65%
Flax	54.2%
Camelina	38.7%
Hemp	17–19%
Walnut	12.9%
Canola	9.1%
Wheat germ	7.8%
Soy	7.7%

Any specific oil's omega-3 content is subject to variation, of course, depending on the soil in which the plant grew and how much sun and rain it received.

We will now take a look at each of these oils individually. The dosage indicated for each oil is the one necessary to meet the body's basic needs, or the daily recommended dosage. A therapeutic dosage would be higher.

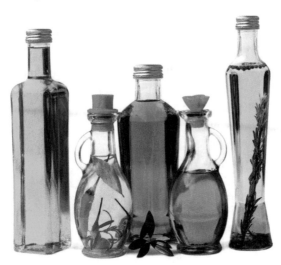

The vegetable oils described in this chapter are the ones that are richest in omega-3s.

Perilla Oil

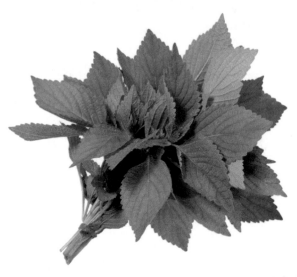

Perilla (*Perilla frutescens*), also known as shiso, is a plant from the mint family that is native to Asia (Japan, China, and Korea). It grows best in full sunlight in areas with high humidity. It has been used for centuries for medicinal purposes, with both internal and external applications, especially for countering allergies and inflammation.

The oil obtained from perilla seeds is extremely rich in omega-3s. Its omega-3 concentration is 65 percent, the highest rate of any source today. This means that you don't need much perilla oil to meet the daily requirements of 2 grams of omega-3s; a dosage of 3 to 4 grams of the oil is sufficient. Achieving such a small dosage is easy with capsules. Using capsules has the added advantage of preventing prolonged contact of the oil with air, which will keep it from becoming rancid.

Dosage:
Take 2 or 3 capsules twice a day, with water. The oil content of the capsules will vary between manufacturers, of course, so be sure to refer to the product label and instructions.

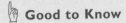

☝ Good to Know

To get the full benefit of omega-3 supplements, take them with a meal that includes fats, as the bile the body releases to digest the fats encourages the assimilation of omega-3s.

Flaxseed Oil

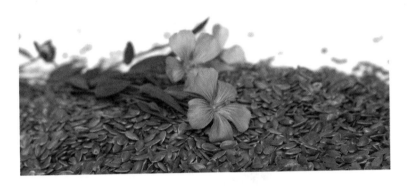

The flax plant (*Linum usitatissimum*) grows to between 1 and 2 feet in height and bears pretty light blue flowers. Humans have cultivated flax for millennia for its textile fibers and its seeds. These seeds are about 30 to 40 percent oil, of which 54 percent are omega-3s. In other words 100 grams of flaxseed oil contains 54 grams of omega-3s. Ingestion of 1 teaspoon of this oil is therefore enough to meet the recommended daily dosage of 2 grams of omega-3s.

Early studies on flaxseed oil suggested that it could be hepatotoxic and impair liver function. However, later studies have disproved these assumptions. It should not be heated, though, or allowed to go rancid. This is why flaxseed oil is only sold in small bottles or in capsule form. The bottles should be of opaque glass in order to protect their contents from the harmful effects of light, and you should store the bottle in the refrigerator after opening.

And, of course, flaxseed oil should never be used for cooking but only consumed raw.

You can also obtain flaxeed's omega-3s by eating the seeds. A hundred grams of flaxseeds contains 40 grams of oil, 20 grams of which are omega-3s. A 10-gram serving of seeds (roughly 2 teaspoons) therefore fulfills the 2-gram omega-3 daily requirement. This method of dosing, however, assumes that the body will assimilate all the omega-3s. For this to happen, you should not ingest the seeds whole but should grind them or let them steep overnight in a glass of water before ingesting them. Another option is to chew them thoroughly before swallowing them.

Dosage:
Oil: Take 1 teaspoon a day.
Seeds: Take 10 grams (2 teaspoons) a day.
Capsules: Take two 1-gram capsules daily.

☝ Good to Know

Doctor Kousmine recommends thoroughly emulsifying flaxseed oil with cottage cheese or fromage blanc. The tiny drops of oil this produces are much more easily assimilated by the body.

The flaxseed oil we are discussing here is food grade and not the same as that used in oil painting (which is toxic and contains no omega-3s). The food-grade oil is sold in health food stores.

Camelina Oil

The camelina plant (*Camelina sativa*) is native to central Europe. Its early growth is characterized by a ring of leaves that cover the ground and prevent weeds from growing. Its stalks can grow as

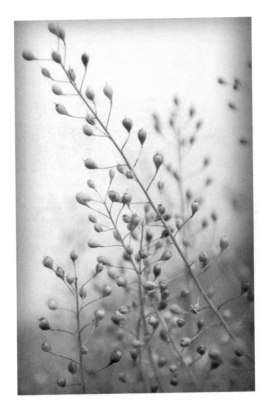

high as 4 feet. They are so stiff that they can be used as a trellis for other plants, such as pea vines. The flowers grow in clusters. Once fertilized they produce capsules containing tiny seeds. Camelina is fairly unknown today, but it was used extensively in the past for its oil by many peoples, including, notably, the Celts.

The contents of camelina seeds are almost entirely lipids, 39 percent of which are omega-3s. Because of this high concentration, camelina has recently regained some of its popularity as an agricultural crop. Just ½ tablespoon of oil fulfills the body's daily requirement for omega-3s. The oil can also be used as a culinary oil, although its high price naturally limits its use.

Dosage:
Take ½ tablespoon a day.

Hempseed Oil

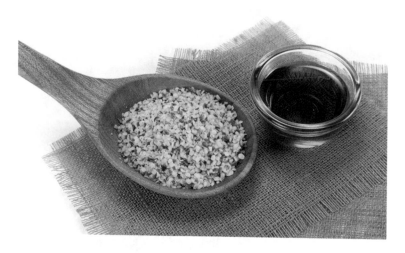

The hemp plant (*Cannabis sativa*) grows from 6 to 10 feet high and features a profusion of handsome, finely notched leaves. A native of Asia, it is now cultivated almost everywhere in the world. Its stalks provide extremely tough fibers that can be used in the production of rope, canvas, paper, and so on. The leaves and flowering tops of some varieties are rich sources of tetrahydrocannabinol (THC) and are used as a drug (marijuana and hashish). The seeds are used to produce oil. The oil we discuss here is produced from the seeds of food-grade hemp and do not contain THC.

Hempseed oil is around 17 to 19 percent omega-3s. One tablespoon (10 grams) therefore meets the body's daily requirement of this nutrient. Though it can be used as a culinary oil—it has a hazelnut-like flavor—its high price naturally limits its use. Hempseed oil is also sold in capsule form.

Dosage:
Oil: Take 1 tablespoon a day
Capsules: Follow the manufacturer's recommended dosage.

English Walnut Oil

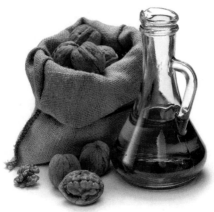

The English walnut tree (*Juglans regia*) is common throughout Europe, and its nuts yield an oil that is between 10 and 13 percent omega-3s. The body's daily requirement for omega-3s can be met by 20 grams of this oil, which comes to 2 tablespoons.

Because of its affordability, walnut oil is a good culinary oil. It is often used to make salad dressings, to which it gives a nutty flavor. However, its acidifying properties are such that it is not recommended for anyone suffering from an acid/alkaline imbalance—in other words, someone whose cellular terrain is acidic.

Dosage:
Take 2 tablespoons a day.

Canola Oil

The canola plant (*Brassica napus*) grows to more than 3 feet in height, and its flowering tops produce tiny, bright yellow flowers. The seeds render 40 percent of their weight in oil. This oil was once considered to be dangerous for humans and its sale was prohibited. But the study (on rats) that had brought it under suspicion of being toxic was later debunked. Today, canola oil is recognized as a high-grade food oil and is popular around the world.

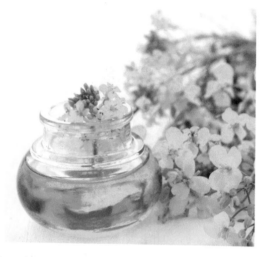

Canola oil is 9 percent omega-3s. Two tablespoons of this oil will fulfill the body's daily minimum requirement for omega-3s.

Canola oil is also quite inexpensive. It can be eaten daily in large quantities in salad dressings, drizzled over steamed vegetables, or in other dishes. Just remember that it retains its omega-3 content only so long as it isn't cooked.

Dosage:
Take 2 tablespoons a day.

Wheat Germ Oil

Wheat germ—the part of the seed from which the plant germinates—is 10 percent oil. This is a fairly small proportion, but this oil contains two valuable nutrients. The first and best

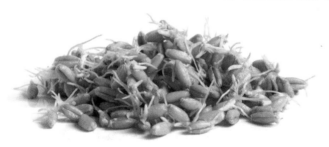

known of the two is a liposoluble vitamin: vitamin E (27 mg per 100 grams of oil). Along with spirulina wheat germ is the richest source of vitamin E. The second nutrient is omega-3s. The oil obtained by pressing wheat germ provides 7.8 grams of omega-3s per 100 grams of oil.

To meet the body's daily requirement for omega-3s, it is therefore necessary to consume 2 to 3 tablespoons of wheat germ oil. This not only is a fairly onerous burden (this oil is not cheap) but is one that is difficult to tolerate physiologically. The oil's high vitamin E content makes it a highly stimulating, even agitating substance—and this is when taken in the normally recommended dose of 1 tablespoon. You wouldn't, therefore, attempt to use wheat germ oil as your sole means of meeting your daily omega-3 requirement. But it can be a valuable supplement for those who are seeking to increase their intake of both omega-3s and vitamin E.

Dosage:
Oil: Take 1 tablespoon a day.
Capsules: Follow the manufacturer's recommended dosage.

Soy Oil

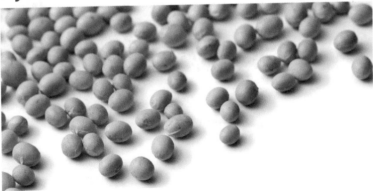

Soy (*Glycine max*) is native to the Far East, where it once grew wild, but it is now cultivated intensively in warm regions around the globe because of its high protein content (35 percent, or twice as much as meat). Soybeans are eaten as is or converted into soy milk or tofu. They were once a mainstay of Eastern diets and have become an increasingly significant part of the Western diet. The beans are also quite high in lipids (22 percent), 7.7 percent of which are omega-3s. Soybean oil is usually quite inexpensive and can be used generously in salad dressings and other dishes. The body's daily requirements for omega-3s can be met with 3 tablespoons of the oil.

Dosage:
Take 3 tablespoons a day.

THE HARMFUL EFFECTS OF TOO MUCH OMEGA-3
It is difficult to have an excess of this nutrient. If one does occur, its effects are:

- Lowered immune system function
- Excessive thinning of the blood
- A reduction of blood sugar levels

⚶

The oils discussed above do not include many of the culinary oils that are popular today. Their omega-3 content is, in fact, quite low, as shown by the table below.

OILS WITH A LOW OMEGA-3 CONTENT	
Oil	Omega-3 Content
Corn oil	0.93%
Olive oil	0.85%
Peanut oil	0.50%
Sunflower oil	0.50%
Grapeseed oil	0.48%
Squash/pumpkin seed oil	0.48%
Safflower oil	0.47%

Their weak concentration of omega-3s means that it would be necessary, for example, to eat 40 tablespoons of sunflower oil to meet the body's daily requirement for omega-3s. A quantity this great would be impossible to digest and cause violent digestive upset. This does not mean that these oils are to be avoided, for they contain other nutrients that are just as valuable for the body—omega-6s, for example.

The current infatuation with omega-3s has pushed omega-6s into the background. These latter are sometimes viewed as being of secondary importance, if not somewhat harmful. It is certainly true that omega-6s do not possess anti-inflammatory virtues, but they play a valuable role in the production of many molecules that are essential for the body. They are the nutrients in mind when people speak of the benefits of vitamin F. See page 152 for more discussion of omega-6s.

Animal Sources of Omega-3s

Omega-3s do not come only from plants; some types of animal flesh have a quite high omega-3 content. This is true of fatty fish living in the cold waters of the northern seas: salmon, herring, mackerel, and, to a lesser extent, tuna. Fish from warmer waters that have high levels of omega-3s include anchovies and sardines. Freshwater rainbow trout also contain good amounts of this valuable nutrient.

? Did You Know?

Because of their high levels of unsaturated fatty acids, fish fats have a soft, rather than solid, consistency. This is why it is more common to speak of fish oil than fish fat.

Fish do not produce omega-3s themselves, but the plankton and algae they consume do. The fish store these omega-3s in their tissues or, to be more specific, in the fats contained in their tissues. As small fish are eaten by larger fish, the omega-3s are passed up and concentrated in the food chain.

The current ongoing interest in omega-3s of marine origin was triggered when studies were performed to understand why the Inuit people of Greenland stayed healthy despite the preponderance of fatty foods (fish, seal, and whale meat) and, thanks to their almost perpetually ice-covered environment, the dearth of plants in their diet. The cardiovascular problems and inflammations that should be prevalent, at first glance, because of their almost exclusive consumption of meat and fish are at most a rare occurrence. The answer to this mystery lay in the rich supplies of omega-3s in their diet, which, as precursors for anti-inflammatory prostaglandins, protect them from inflammation and thickening of the blood.

The 2 grams of omega-3s the body needs daily are in fact easily supplied by relatively small portions of these fish, as shown by the table below. Thus, a large supply of omega-3s for the purpose of fighting inflammation can be provided by regular consumption of these fish.

QUANTITY OF FISH NECESSARY TO PROVIDE 2 GRAMS OF OMEGA-3S

- 80 grams of Atlantic mackerel
- 100 grams of Atlantic salmon (farm raised)
- 120 grams of canned pink salmon
- 120 grams of Pacific or Atlantic herring
- 140 grams of Pacific mackerel
- 200 grams of rainbow trout (farm raised)
- 200 grams of sardines
- 260 grams of canned tuna

Fish Oil

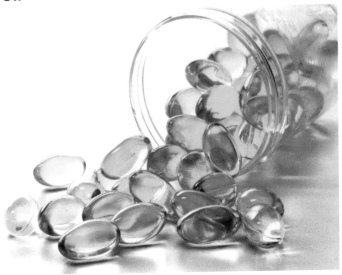

Some people do not like fish or do not wish to eat it every day. Does this mean they cannot enjoy the benefits of marine-sourced omega-3s? No, because fish oil is also available in the form of capsules. They are produced as a by-product of commercial fishing. After the various prime cuts of the fish have been taken, the meat that remains is subjected to a special process that extracts the oil, which is then put into capsules.

Make sure that you do not mistake these oils for the cod liver and halibut liver oils that are prescribed for their vitamin A and D content.

Fish oil capsules most commonly contain 1 gram of fish oil, which works out to 300 grams of omega-3s. It is therefore necessary to take two capsules at least three times a day to meet the body's daily requirement.

Fish oil is also sold in small bottles. To reduce its strong fishy odor, it is often combined with lemon or orange scent. This form may be preferred when substantial amounts are necessary for therapeutic purposes, so as to avoid having to take an excessive number of capsules.

High doses of fish oil can cause little inconveniences such as softening of the stools, nausea, and lingering odors or regurgitations with a fishy taste. To avoid this last drawback, it is advisable to take the capsules at the beginning of a meal.

Dosage:

Oil: Follow the manufacturer's instructions.

Capsules: Dosages may vary depending on the product, but in general, take 2 capsules three times daily, before meals. Note: Fish oil capsules are often quite large. Before buying them, make sure that you will be able to swallow them!

Contraindications: Avoid marine-sourced omega-3s if you are allergic to fish.

The Omega-6–Omega-3 Relationship

The properties of omega-6 fatty acids are directly opposite to those of omega-3s. Omega-6s cause inflammation, are vasoconstrictors, and thicken the blood, whereas omega-3s reduce or prevent inflammation, are vasodilators, and thin the blood. Both types of fatty acids are useful to the body, but they need to be supplied to it in appropriate proportions. Ideally, it seems that this ratio should be five parts omega-6s to one part omega-3s. In practice though, the ratio provided by the Western diet is more typically ten or even thirty to one, thus providing a clear excess of omega-6s to the body.

The correction of this ratio can be achieved by reducing consumption of foods rich in omega-6s (meats, dairy products, and certain vegetable oils) and increasing consumption of those that are rich in omega-3s (canola and flaxseed oils, fish, almonds, walnuts, et cetera).

Plant Sources of Gamma-Linolenic Acid

The oils produced by evening primrose and borage are often recommended as treatment for inflammation because they encourage the production of anti-inflammatory prostaglandins. They do not contain any omega-3s, however. How then can they have anti-inflammatory properties?

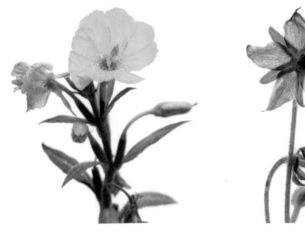
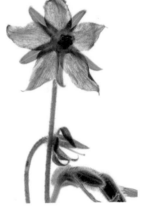

Evening primrose   *Borage*

Omega-3 fatty acids are not the only substances from which the body manufactures anti-inflammatory prostaglandins. It can also produce them from one of the omega-6s: linoleic acid. (Linoleic acid—which is an omega-6—should not be confused with linolenic acid, which is an omega-3.)

Linoleic acid can be found in abundance in vegetable oils, almonds, egg yolks, and other dietary staples. However, the body must first transform linoleic acid into gamma-linolenic acid (GLA) before it can create anti-inflammatory prostaglandins from it. This transformation occurs easily in people who enjoy good health. It is much more difficult, if it occurs at all, in people who are sick—who ironically are the individuals who need it most. The degraded state of their cellular terrain impedes the various mechanisms that must be brought together in order for this transformation to occur.

☝ Good to Know

Many different fatty acids are classified as omega-6s. The primary ones are:

- Linoleic acid
- Arachidonic acid
- Gamma-linolenic acid

The delta-6 desaturase enzyme is key to transforming linoleic acid to GLA, and it must be supported by adequate levels of zinc, magnesium, vitamin B_6, and biotin. A patient who is ill or otherwise deficient may lack these nutrients. Moreover, the enzyme can be inhibited by many elements that, in our day, are often present in the body, especially for those who are ill. Among these inhibiting factors we can include saturated fats, cholesterol, alcohol, certain viruses, chemical carcinogens, ionizing radiation, and a deficiency of insulin.

If these inhibiting factors or deficiencies are present, the body will be unable to convert linoleic acid into GLA, and this substance will in turn be unavailable for the creation of anti-inflamatory prostaglandins.

The obstacle posed by the nontransformation of linoleic acid into GLA can, however, be overcome. In fact, nature provides already-formed GLA. Two plants in particular carry an abundance of this substance in their seeds: evening primrose and borage. When the oil extracted from their seeds is ingested, the body no longer has to rely on the first transformation in order to obtain GLA; it receives its supply directly. The body's only task, then, is to transform the GLA into anti-inflammatory prostaglandins.

THE TRANSFORMATION OF LINOLEIC ACID INTO ANTI-INFLAMMATORY PROSTAGLANDINS

Stage 1 • Cis-Linoleic Acid

↓

Delta-6 desaturase enzyme necessary for the transition to stage 2

↓

Helped by

Zinc, magnesium, vitamin B_6, biotin (vitamin B_8)

↓

Inhibited by

Trans fatty acids   Excess of alcohol
Saturated fats   Senility
Cholesterol   Some viruses
Zinc deficiency   Chemical carcinogens
Insulin deficiency   Ionzing radiation

↓

Stage 2 • Gamma-Linolenic Acid

Evening primrose and borage oil start here

↓

Stage 3 • Dihomo-Gamma-Linolenic Acid

Helped by

Vitamins C and B_3

↓

Stage 4 • Anti-Inflammatory Prostaglandins

Based on *Les 5 piliers de la santé* [The 5 Pillars of Health] by P. G. Besson, A. Denjean, and P. Keros (St.-Julien-en-Genevois, France: Editions Jouvence, 1993).

Evening Primrose Oil

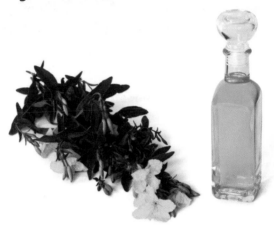

Evening primrose (*Oenothera biennis*) is native to North America, where it was used for medicinal purposes by Native Americans. It spread into Europe starting in the seventeenth century. Its yellow flowers have the peculiar feature of opening in the evening and closing during the day; for this reason it's sometimes also known as "evening star" and "queen of the night." The flower opens over a period of several minutes and is a spectacular sight to observe.

Evening primrose seeds produce an oil that ranges from 8 to 11 percent GLA. Its seeds are tiny but it has a great volume of them. The quantity of oil that can be extracted from them is still low, hence its high price.

Evening primrose oil will go rancid very quickly upon contact with air (in less than a half hour), which is why it is primarily sold in capsule form. The contents of the capsules vary from 500 mg to 1000 mg or even 1300 mg. The manufacturer's instructions provide the correct dosage; generally speaking, it is necessary to take two 500 mg capsules with water three times a day, at mealtimes.

Dosage:
Follow the manufacturer's instructions.

Borage Oil

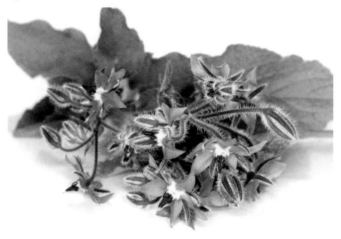

The borage plant (*Borago officinalis*) can grow as high as 2 feet. Its stalks and leaves bristle with little hairs, which gives it a somewhat diaphanous appearance. Its blue flowers, which have five petals in the shape of a star, are small and droop down. Borage multiplies readily in gardens and along paths and roadsides. While it was once used for food (its leaves can be cooked or used as salad greens), today it is grown primarily for its medicinal properties.

Borage's primary property is that it is sudorific (encourages perspiration). According to some experts, this property is responsible for its name: in Arabic *bou* means "father" and *rash* means "sweat," thus "father of sweat." Borage is also a diuretic and a laxative. But the property that concerns us here is the one contained in its seeds. Like those of the evening primrose, they are tiny but contain an oil that is rich in gamma-linolenic acid. It averages between 20 and 26 percent of the oil.

In order to preserve borage oil from contact with air, which will encourage rancidity and destroy its valuable properties, borage oil is sold in capsule form, generally with a content of 500 mg.

Dosage:

Take 2 capsules two times daily (or follow the manufacturer's dosage instruction).

ALKALINE SUPPLEMENTS

We now need to examine the second kind of dietary supplements that can help calm inflammation: alkaline minerals. The alkaline minerals have an anti-inflammatory effect by virtue of the fact they are capable of neutralizing excess acids in the tissues. These acids are aggressive and irritating substances. When acid levels in the tissues are too high, the acids will trigger inflammations or intensify those that are present for other reasons (due to infections or allergies, for example).

Normally the acid substances in our body are counterbalanced by an equal amount of alkaline substances. This is what we mean when we speak of an acid-alkaline balance. Far too often, though, this balance is broken and the terrain becomes acidified. This condition is described as acidosis. The main cause of this acidification is the quantitatively higher consumption of acidifying foods (meats, grains, white sugar, fats, wine, coffee) than alkalizing foods (cooked and raw vegetables, greens, potatoes, almonds, bananas, sweet fruits). Other causes are insufficient oxygenation, stress, overwork, and lack of sleep.*

Acidity in the cellular terrain is itself a cause of inflammation, and it should be considered when no external cause for the inflammation can be determined. The reason is the easily seen aggressive nature of acids. When you chomp into a stalk of rhubarb or an acidic fruit like a lemon or a green apple, for

---

*To learn more, see my book *The Acid-Alkaline Diet for Optimum Health: Restore Your Health by Creating pH Balance in Your Diet* (Rochester, Vt.: Healing Arts Press, 2006).

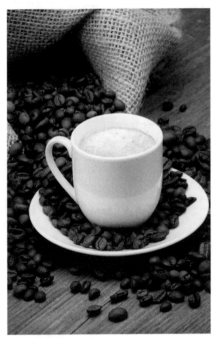

Acidifying foods like coffee should be balanced with alkalizing foods.

example, a defensive reaction instantly takes place to counter the attack of the acid: the face and mouth contract, and excessive amounts of saliva are released to dilute the irritating agent. Just how aggressive the acid of a lemon can be is shown by an experiment that consists of placing a slice of lemon on a piece of polished marble. After several days the smooth surface of the marble will have been eaten into and become rough and pitted.

Another example: You can take advantage of the aggressive nature of the acids in vinegar to dissolve chalky deposits on the bottom of pots or bathtubs. The experiment of submerging a piece of meat in a cola soda is well known. After a day or two, the piece of meat will be dissolved completely by the acids of the cola (and, in fact, cola was once much more acidic than it is today). Anyone who has ever gotten lemon juice in a fresh cut on their hand can verify the extremely painful sting.

Acids act in identical fashion inside the human body. They attack the tissues, irritating and eating away at them, and eventually destroying them. When this occurs on the skin, we see red patches, itching, and eczema. When it occurs in the joints, we see pain, swelling, and attacks of tendinitis. Acids are responsible for neuritis in the nerves, as well as neuralgia, sciatica, and so on. The tissues become red, warm, painful, and swollen. All the different symptoms of inflammation are present. The organs, too, are vulnerable to inflammatory disorders caused by excessive acids in the body. These disorders are engendered by acids we consume or those the body produces in excess when overworked or subjected to stress.

An acidified terrain is a pro-inflammatory terrain.

Inflammations due to acidification can be treated by removing acids from the terrain. The deacidification process is achieved through a generous ingestion of alkaline minerals, which neutralize the excess acids by "buffering" them—in other words by combining with them. An alkaline that combines with an acid produces a neutral salt. The supply of alkaline minerals can be assured either by following an alkaline diet or by taking alkaline supplements. These steps can be combined in order to hasten the deacidification of the terrain.

The Alkaline Diet

This is a diet that contains a higher proportion of alkalizing foods than acidifying ones. Such a diet can be established by referring to the lists of alkalizing and acidifying foods provided below.

An alkaline-heavy diet will provide not just enough alkaline substances to neutralize the acidifying elements in your daily diet, but a surplus of these substances that the body can use to neutralize acids stored in its cellular terrain. The further this neutralization progresses, the less acid remains in the terrain and the more inflammation will be soothed.

⚠ Caution!

Acidifying foods should not be entirely eliminated from the diet, as they contain basic nutrients, notably those that provide the body with essential proteins.

ALKALIZING FOODS

- Potatoes
- Green vegetables, raw or cooked: greens, lettuce, green beans, cabbage, and so on
- Colored vegetables: carrots, beets, and so on (except tomatoes)
- Milk, powdered milk, well-drained quark cheese, cream
- Bananas
- Almonds (and almond milk), Brazil nuts, chestnuts
- Dried fruits (except apricots)
- Alkaline mineral waters

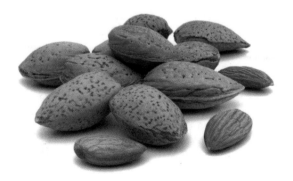

ACIDIFYING FOODS

- Meat, poultry, cold cuts, meat extracts, fish
- Cheese (strong cheeses are more acidic than mild ones)
- Animal fats
- Vegetable oils, especially peanut and refined oils
- Grains (whole or not), including oats, and especially millet
- Bread, pasta, cereals, and grain-based foods
- Legumes: peanuts, soybeans, white beans, favas, and so forth
- Refined white sugar
- Sweets: syrup, pastries, chocolate, candies, jam, and so on
- All nuts except the ones named above
- Coffee, tea, cocoa, wine

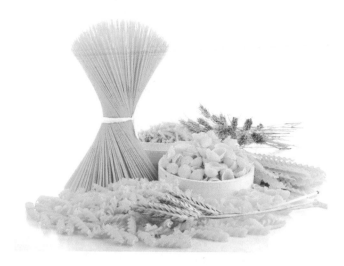

WEAKLY ACIDIC FOODS

These foods are alkalizing for individuals who easily metabolize weak acids, but they are acidifying for others. The first group should increase their consumption of them, while the second should reduce their consumption, if not eliminate them completely from their diet, at least temporarily.

- Whey that is more than several hours old (thus yogurt, curdled milk, kefir, unstrained cottage cheese, fromage blanc, and so on)
- Unripe fruits (the less ripe the fruit, the more acid it contains)
- Acidic fruits: berries, currants, black currants, raspberries, and so on
- Citrus fruits: lemon, grapefruit, orange, and so on
- Tart apples, cherries, plums, and apricots
- Large amounts of sweet fruit
- Acidic vegetables: tomatoes, rhubarb, watercress, sorrel
- Sauerkraut and other fermented vegetables
- Fruit juices, lemon juice
- Sweet carbonated beverages like colas and sodas
- Honey
- Vinegar

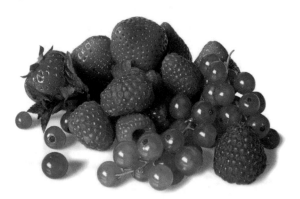

Alkaline Mineral Supplements

Alkaline supplements consist of a blend of different alkaline minerals like calcium, potassium, magnesium, manganese, iron, sodium, and so forth. Supplements contain these minerals in a form that is easily assimilated and in balanced proportions.

They are manufactured as both powders and tablets. These supplements make it possible to easily obtain a concentrated supply of alkaline substances.

👆 **Good to Know**

The pH scale measures the acidity of various substances, indicating the degree of a substance's acidity or alkalinity. The measuring scale goes from 0 to 14.

- A pH of 7 is neutral.
- A pH of 7 to 1 reflects an increasing amount of acidity.
- A pH of 7 to 14 reflects an increasing amount of alkalinity.

The most effective dosage for alkaline supplements is whatever amount is sufficient to yield a urine pH of 7. This pH is considered normal for urine. The urine of a person suffering from an overly acidified terrain will have a lower pH because his or her body is attempting to rid itself of the excess acids. The urine in this case may veer toward a pH of 6.5 or lower. The lower the pH, the more acidified the terrain.

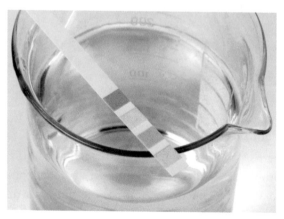

A strip of litmus paper can be used to test the pH of urine.

Urine pH can be measured with the help of litmus paper, which is available in most pharmacies. To effectively measure urine pH, test your urine every time you urinate over a two- to three-day period.

By providing the body with an abundance of alkaline substances, you give it the materials it needs to deacidify the terrain. The elimination of the excess acids will bring about a gradual reduction and elimination of endogenous inflammatory disorders.

While the removal of excess acids from the depths of the terrain can take several months, improvement in symptoms can be felt after just a few days. For example, the pain caused by inflammation in acidified individuals can rapidly diminish in intensity, if not disappear outright. In fact, the rapidity of the analgesic effect almost always comes as a surprise to the affected individuals.

We've discussed deacidification and this analgesic effect in terms of endogenous inflammatory conditions—those arising from internal factors, namely an acidic terrain—but it so happens that this action can also be beneficially put to use in treating inflammations caused by exogenous factors—in other words those due to infection or to contact with allergens. It is a fact that these inflammations usually take place in an already acidified terrain.

☝ Good to Know

An inflammation caused by exogenous factors is often in addition to one already established by an acidic terrain. The latent aggression of the acids joins with the isolated attack of the germs or allergens. The exogenous inflammation is aggravated and intensified by the presence of acids. Furthermore, the exogenous inflammation will produce acids on its own due to the overall acceleration of the metabolism, the destruction of the tissues, and the battle waged by the lymphocytes against the invaders.

One part of the treatment of any inflammation, then, whether endogenous or exogenous, should logically consist of countering the acidic nature of the terrain by taking alkaline supplements. Take enough powder or tablets (three times a day, with water) as is necessary to obtain a urine pH of 7.

CONCLUSION

Nutrition is being increasingly recognized as its own separate therapy. Two examples of the soundness of this opinion can be found in the use of omega-3s and alkaline supplements to combat inflammatory diseases.

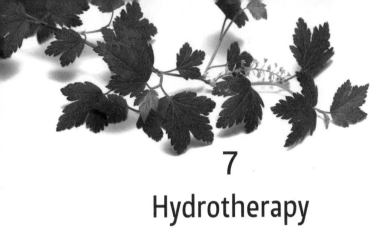

7
Hydrotherapy
The Anti-Inflammatory Effect of Cold Water

Hydrotherapy is a treatment that consists of applying either cold or hot water on the body's surface. The site and duration of the application vary in accordance with the patient's needs. The purpose of these applications is to stimulate necessary physiological exchanges when they are insufficient or to slow them down when they are too intense. The results of the treatment manifest not just on the surface of the body but also in its depths, in the blood capillaries, muscles, and organs.

With respect to the effects of hot hydrotherapy, as a quick summary I can say that the heat warms what is cold, dilates what is contracted, accelerates what has slowed down, and intensifies blood circulation. If you consider it closely, its effects are identical to those of inflammation: heat (the increase in body temperature), tumescence (swelling of the tissues), redness (intensification of blood flow), and pain (when it becomes too hot).

Knowing this, it is easy to grasp the value that therapeutic

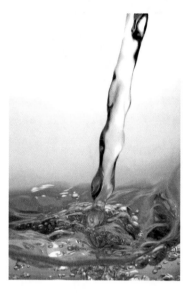

The benefits of cold hydrotherapy for inflammation have long been proven.

applications of cold water can have. Cold cools down what is hot, contracts what is dilated, slows down what is moving too fast, and soothes pain. More specifically, the contact of cold water with a hot, inflamed zone naturally causes it to lose its heat; in other words it cools down, which causes the capillaries to tighten up. This vasoconstrictive effect reduces blood circulation to the region, which will cause it to lose its red color. The vasoconstriction also causes the tissues to tighten up, which expels the plasma stored there and thereby reduces swelling in that zone. The cold also "anesthetizes" the nerves, reducing their sensitivity as well as their ability to transmit signals, thereby yielding an analgesic effect.

THE LIMITS OF COLD HYDROTHERAPY

While cold hydrotherapy has anti-inflammatory effects, it cannot counter all the disorders caused by inflammation. In fact, in some situations cold hydrotherapy is contraindicated, as the cold water can actually aggravate the patient's condition.

Human beings are warm-blooded creatures, with a fixed internal temperature of 98.6°F. Slight deviations above or below this mark are possible, but normally they are minimal (a variance of only a couple degrees). Moreover, the body is always working to maintain this ideal temperature. An application of cold water threatens the body's thermic balance, compelling it to react and call upon its own forces. Here we encounter the first delicate point of cold water applications: The amount of cold applied to the body should not outstrip the body's abilities to neutralize it. If too much cold is applied, the body will overexert itself in response and become weaker. The strength it could use to oppose germs, allergens, or other irritants will be reduced; they will then gain the upper hand and the inflammation will worsen.

For this reason the intensity of coldness in the hydrotherapy treatment must be very precisely monitored. To begin usually the water should be cool (around 77°F) as opposed to cold (40°), and the length of time for which it is applied should be limited (one to two minutes, rather than fifteen minutes). It is also

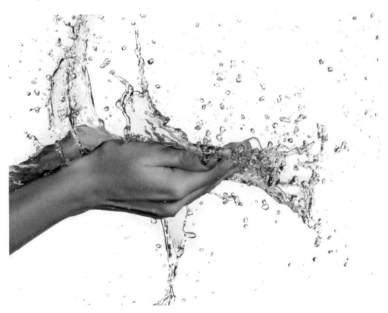

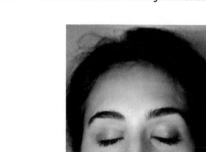

The nose does not react effectively against the cold.

important to confine the application to just the part of the body that is inflamed and painful.

However, even when taking all these precautions, some organs are simply not capable of reacting effectively against the cold, and they should not be subject to cold hydrotherapy. These organs include the nose, the lungs, the kidneys, the bladder, the stomach, and the intestines. But why are these organs particularly vulnerable to the cold? Few explanations have been provided, but it could be because these organs are hollow—that is, they have thin walls containing a large cavity. The walls of the lungs, for example, are formed by the rib cage and pleura, while those of the intestines are made up of very thin mucous membranes. As a result these organs may not have enough volume and blood to react effectively. Furthermore, they are constantly losing heat to their cavity.

THE BENEFITS OF COLD HYDROTHERAPY

It is an entirely different story for those organs that are heavily irrigated by blood vessels (such as the skin and muscles), whose cavity is filled with blood (such as blood vessels), or that are firmly surrounded by flesh and blood vessels (such as bones, joints, tendons, and nerves). Cold hydrotherapeutic applications are highly beneficial for these organs.

COLD HYDROTHERAPY EFFECTS ON ORGANS	
Beneficial	**Contraindicated**
Skin	Respiratory tract
Muscles	Digestive tract
Joints	Kidneys
Tendons	Bladder
Nerves	

If, instead of considering the organs, we concentrate on the diseases and disorders that can or cannot benefit from cold hydrotherapy, we come up with the following list:

COLD HYDROTHERAPY EFFECTS ON DISEASES AND DISORDERS	
Beneficial	**Contraindicated**
Insect stings	Colds
Burns	Bronchitis
Itching	Nephritis
Eczema	Cystitis
Aching muscles	Enteritis
Neuritis	Colitis
Tendinitis	Prostatitis

COLD HYDROTHERAPY EFFECTS ON DISEASES AND DISORDERS (continued)	
Beneficial	**Contraindicated**
Sciatica	
Phlebitis	
Hemorrhoids	
Conjunctivitis	
Sties	
Dental pain	

As in all other fields, the general rules of hydrotherapy must be adapted for each individual case. Though nerve inflammation (neuritis, sciatica, toothache) and the pain it causes can be soothed by cold hydrotherapeutic applications for some people, for other people that problem will not be relieved by these treatments but will be aggravated. It is rarely possible to know in advance how an individual will react to this treatment; it has to be discovered by trying it. So it is extremely important when starting such treatment to pay very close attention to the patient's reaction, so that you will quickly detect any signs indicating that it is not working.

SOME COLD HYDROTHERAPY APPLICATIONS

When I use the term "cold water," I mean water whose temperature is sufficiently lower than that of the body to be felt as cold. As normal body temperature is 98.6°F, water is considered lukewarm until it falls to a temperature of around 80°F to 81°F. It is considered cool at around 72°F and cold at 59°F. It is considered very cold at around 44°F. At 32°F it turns to ice, which can also be used for the purpose of hydrotherapy.

The lower the temperature of the water, the shorter its application to the body should be. A person can bathe in 77°F water for many minutes at a time, as when swimming in a pool or at the seaside. In contrast icy water or ice cubes should remain in contact with the body for no more than a few minutes.

Here are three cold hydrotherapy techniques that have proven effective in treating inflammation.

Bag of Ice

Because it employs ice, this application has a powerful effect that brings inflammation to a screeching halt, at least momentarily. The icy cold anesthetizes the area and reduces or even eliminates the pain caused by the inflammation.

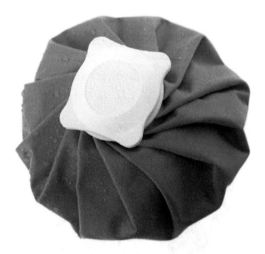

Indications: Insect sting, headache, contusion, toothache, joint pain, hemorrhoids, phlebitis, tendinitis

Materials: Whole ice cubes or shards (use a hammer), a plastic bag, a protective cloth

Preparation: Place the ice cubes in the plastic bag. Use enough ice to cover the entire area needing treatment, but no more.

Application: Place a protective cloth over the affected area to protect the skin from the ice. Fold the cloth as needed, in accordance with the sensitivity of the individual receiving the cold treatment. Place the poultice on the cloth.

Duration: Apply for one to three minutes; base the duration on the patient's reaction to the treatment.

Frequency: Repeat this application two or three times during the day, or more often if needed.

Cold Water Compress

The effects of this compress are similar to those of the bag of ice, but much less intense, and thus less profound and of shorter duration. The compress will quickly lose its temperature once it enters in contact with the heat of the inflammation, which is not the case for the bag of ice. However, the specific advantages of the compress are its less violent nature and the possibility of applying it for longer periods of time.

Indications: Conjunctivitis, eczema, hives, itching, allergic

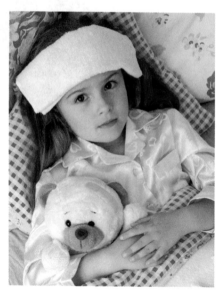

reactions in the skin and eyes, thrush, athlete's foot, neuritis, joint pain, phlebitis, tonsillitis, sore throat

Material: A bowl of cold water, ice cubes, a cloth large enough to fold several times and then cover the entire area needing treatment

Preparation: Place the ice cubes in the cold water. When the water has attained the desired temperature, dip the compress into it, and lightly squeeze it to wring out excess water.

Application: Place the water-soaked compress over the inflamed zone.

Duration: Remove the compress before it becomes warm, dip it again in the cold water, and place it back over the affected area.

Frequency: Repeat the application as often as desired.

Cold Clay Poultice

The density of the support—the clay here—holds the cold temperature longer. A clay poultice will lose its temperature less quickly than the cold water compress described above, for the simple reason that water has less density than clay. This makes it possible to have longer applications, with deeply penetrating effects.

Indications: Acne, abscess, boil, toothache, joint pain, tendinitis

Material: Powdered clay, a bowl of cold water, a wooden spatula or other mixing utensil

Preparation: Using the wooden spatula, blend the powdered clay with the cold water until you obtain a very moist but solid paste. If necessary, you can place the paste in the refrigerator for a few minutes to make it colder.

Application: Spread the clay over the affected area in a layer that is ¼ to ¾ inch thick.

Duration: Leave the poultice in place until it turns lukewarm (which will take thirty minutes or more).

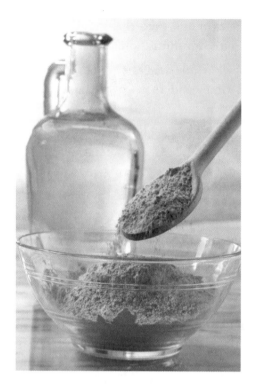

Frequency: Put a new poultice on immediately or after several hours, as desired. Apply two or three poultices a day.

CONCLUSION

Cold hydrotherapy is a simple, effective, inexpensive, and rapid means for calming an inflammation and easing the pain it causes. It can be used as an emergency treatment or as a supplement to other anti-inflammatory treatments.

Directory of Illnesses and Recommended Anti-Inflammatories

Inflammation has many, many manifestations in the body. We've discussed some of these diseases in depth over the preceding pages; others we have only touched on, or have not addressed directly. Nevertheless, just about any inflammatory condition can be treated with the anti-inflammatory plants profiled in chapter 5, complemented by the supplements and techniques outlined in chapters 6 and 7. The listing below identifies the plants that can be used to treat a wide range of inflammatory conditions. The plants are listed in order of their typical effectiveness, beginning with those that are generally most effective in treating the disorder in question.

You can, of course, choose more than one plant to treat an inflammation. You may, in fact, find it especially effective to treat such a condition both internally and externally.

Illness	Suggested Plants for Treatment
Abrasions	Roman chamomile, lavender, lemon eucalyptus, bay laurel, propolis
Abscess	Propolis, lemon eucalyptus, bay laurel, turmeric
Acne	Propolis, lemon eucalyptus, bay laurel, turmeric
Allergies	Black currant, Scotch pine, black spruce, black cumin, birch, English oak
Angioedema	See *Quincke's edema*
Arteritis	Black currant, lemon eucalyptus
Arthritis	Devil's claw, lemon eucalyptus, black currant, meadowsweet, white willow, wintergreen, bay laurel, turmeric, Scotch pine
Asthma	Scotch pine, black spruce, bay laurel, black currant
Back pain	See *lumbago*
Bite (insect)	See *insect sting*
Blepharitis	Eyebright, Roman chamomile
Boil	See *acne*
Bronchitis	Scotch pine, black spruce, bay laurel, propolis, lavender
Burns	See *sunburn*
Canker sores	Black currant, bay laurel, propolis
Cavities (painful)	See *headache*
Colitis	Basil, cumin, bay laurel, black spruce, propolis, Roman chamomile
Common cold	Propolis, bay laurel, black spruce, black currant, eyebright, Scotch pine
Conjunctivitis	Eyebright, Roman chamomile
Cough	Lavender, bay laurel, Scotch pine, black spruce
Cracked lips, skin	Propolis, lavender, Roman chamomile, turmeric
Cystitis	Basil, black currant, propolis, black spruce

Illness	Suggested Plants for Treatment
Dental pain	See *toothache*
Diarrhea	Basil, bay laurel, turmeric, black spruce, propolis
Eczema	Lavender, lemon eucalyptus, bay laurel, Roman chamomile, turmeric, propolis
Enteritis	Basil, black spruce, turmeric, Roman chamomile, bay laurel, propolis, lavender
Epicondylitis	See *tendinitis*
Eye irritation	See *conjunctivitis*
Gastritis	See *heartburn*
Gastroenteritis	Basil, bay laurel, propolis, black spruce, Roman chamomile, turmeric
Gingivitis	Black currant, bay laurel, propolis, lavender, Roman chamomile
Glossitis	See *gingivitis*
Gout	Black currant, meadowsweet, lemon eucalyptus, white willow, birch, black spruce, bay laurel
Headache	Black cumin, wintergreen, lavender
Heartburn	Roman chamomile, basil, bay laurel, propolis
Hemorrhoids	Black currant, lemon eucalyptus
Hives	Black currant, Scotch pine, Roman chamomile, lavender, lemon eucalyptus, bay laurel
Insect sting	Lemon eucalyptus, lavender, propolis, bay laurel
Intestinal irritation	See *enteritis*
Irritable bowel syndrome	Bay laurel, basil, lavender, turmeric, Roman chamomile
Itching	Roman chamomile, lavender, lemon eucalyptus, black currant, bay laurel

Illness	Suggested Plants for Treatment
Keratitis	See *conjunctivitis*
Laryngitis	See *loss of voice*
Loss of voice (aphonia)	Propolis, bay laurel, lavender
Lumbago	Wintergreen, lemon eucalyptus, devil's claw, bay laurel, meadowsweet, white willow
Muscle strain	Wintergreen, lemon eucalyptus, bay laurel, devil's claw
Mycosis	Lemon eucalyptus, bay laurel, propolis, lavender, Roman chamomile
Neuralgia	See *neuritis*
Neuritis	Black currant, basil, bay laurel, wintergreen, lemon eucalyptus, Roman chamomile, meadowsweet, white willow
Osteoarthritis	See *arthritis*
Otitis	Lavender, propolis
Pain (general)	See *arthritis*
Periodontitis	Bay laurel, lavender, propolis, Roman chamomile, black currant
Pharyngitis	See *sore throat*
Phlebitis	Black currant, lemon eucalyptus
Polyarthritis	See *arthritis*
Prostatitis	Black currant, basil, propolis, Scotch pine, black spruce
Pruritis	See *itching*

Illness	Suggested Plants for Treatment
Quincke's edema	Black currant
Rheumatism	See *arthritis*
Rhinitis	See *common cold*
Rhinopharyngitis	See *sore throat*
Shingles	Basil, bay laurel, lemon eucalyptus, wintergreen
Sinusitis	Black spruce, bay laurel, Scotch pine, propolis, lavender
Sore throat	Propolis, lavender, bay laurel, Scotch pine, black spruce
Stomach ulcer	See *heartburn*
Stomatitis	See *gingivitis*
Sty	Eyebright, Roman chamomile
Sunburn	Lavender, Roman chamomile
Tendinitis	Wintergreen, lemon eucalyptus, black currant, meadowsweet, white willow, bay laurel, devil's claw, basil
Tennis elbow	See *tendinitis*
Tonsillitis	Propolis, bay laurel
Toothache	Bay laurel, propolis, Roman chamomile, lavender, black currant
Tracheitis	See *sore throat*
Urethritis	See *cystitis*
Whitlow	Lemon eucalyptus, propolis, bay laurel, lavender, turmeric
Wounds/cuts	Roman chamomile, lavender, propolis

ILLUSTRATION CREDITS

Index

Page numbers in *italics* refer to images.

183

184 ⚹ Index